The Menopause Makeover

The Ultimate Guide to Taking
Control of Your Health and Beauty
During Menopause

STANESS JONEKOS

WITH WENDY KLEIN, M.D.

The Menopause Makeover
ISBN-10: 0-9972150-0-3
ISBN-13: 978-0-9972150-0-7

Jonekos, Staness.
The menopause makeover: the ultimate guide to taking control of your health
and beauty during menopause / Staness Jonekos with Wendy Klein.

Photo credits:
Before Menopause photo by David LaPore
After Menopause photo by Michael Becker
Staness Jonekos author photo by Michael Becker
Wendy Klein, M.D. author photo by Al Wekelo

www.MenopauseMakeover.com

Printed in the U.S.A.

The health and medical information provided in this book is not intended to take the place of advice or treatment from your healthcare professionals. The authors have worked hard to ensure the information provided in this book is timely, accurate and helpful. This information should not be considered medical advice. One should consult with their healthcare provider. The information provided is for general reference purposes only. Always obtain advice from your physician or other qualified health professional before starting any new treatment.

To my husband, Michael, who showed me I was lovable before,
during and after menopause.

This book is dedicated to the women before us who suffered in silence,
and to the women stepping out of the 'menopause closet' today who show
the world it's OK to talk about menopause. Our positive attitude towards
menopause today will pave the path for all women in the future.

Also by Staness Jonekos:

Eat Like a Woman and Never Diet Again
with Marjorie Jenkins, MD, MEHP, FACP

www.EatLikeAWoman.com

All Essential Planner tools, health calculators, additional resources and references are available at www.MenopauseMakeover.com

Contents

Marriage and Menopause?

At forty-seven, I was busy planning my first wedding after thirty years of dating in Los Angeles. It was a joyful time, with the exception of hourly hot flashes, weight gain that made it impossible to pre-order the wedding dress of my choice, and a vagina that was in no mood for a honeymoon. I was desperate to find solutions to my miserable menopause symptoms so I could feel like myself again, and look like the woman my fiancé fell in love with. I prayed my doctor would have a magic pill, but she did not.

I began an urgent quest for answers that would allow me to regain control over my health and beauty before the big wedding day. I needed a Menopause Makeover! There were many books and websites about menopause, but none had an action plan to guide me through the confusing array of treatment options. During my search, I discovered the actual process of planning my wedding held the key to my Menopause Makeover. Managing menopause, for me, was going to take the same amount of effort as planning a wedding.

Since I had less than four months until my wedding, and there were no "menopause makeover" books available, I created a 12-week plan to manage my uninvited wedding guest, menopause. Inspired by my own wedding planner book, which offered succinct information, checklists, to-do lists, and a place to journal, set goals, and track progress, my makeover plan helped me reclaim my health—and my life—in just three months.

I ended up with two planners in my life, one for my wedding and one for my menopause. Marriage and menopause made an odd pair, but the dual planner approach worked! My menopause makeover plan gave me the direction I needed to accomplish my goals in twelve weeks.

Going through menopause was a wake-up call for me. I could no longer ignore my bad eating habits, lack of exercise, and health issues that popped up, such as high blood pressure and fading vision. Most of us are busy with family, career, children, home, and parents, with no time left for ourselves. Menopause will demand your attention. Making a commitment to the 12-Week Menopause Makeover is the first step to taking control of your health and beauty at midlife. It is the key to a new and revitalized you!

MY STORY: WHY I WROTE THIS BOOK

It took forty-six years for true love to find me and just six months for menopause to seize me. And when I said, "I do" to the man of my dreams, I said, "I don't" to hot flashes, a dry vagina and an ever-expanding waistline.

Menopause hit me at full speed. Before getting married, I decided to get a FSH (follicle stimulating hormone) test to determine whether or not I was still fertile. I had been on birth control pills for 25 years. Getting off the pill to get a "true" FSH test sent my body into chaos. Little did I know that over the years, my "natural" state had started shutting down and had entered a stage of menopause. My FSH test result was 72. Generally, any number over 40 mIU/ML indicates that the ovaries are not producing enough estrogen to keep monthly periods normal (see Chapter One for more information).

I was in a state of shock at the results. No one told me how dramatic it would be to experience "the change." When my mother's hormones started changing in her forties, she had a hysterectomy and immediately began taking a hormone therapy drug called Premarin, an oral form of estrogen. My family never saw any "changes" in my mother, other than that she seemed happier. All of my friends got married much earlier than I did, had their children, and were nowhere close to menopause. Feeling terribly unprepared, I entered one of the most challenging phases in my life, getting married and "getting" menopause alone.

As any bride knows, the day you get married is the day you want to feel like a princess. We spend months preparing for the big event. Beautifying, pampering, slipping into wedding gowns, hoping to discover the one dress that makes us feel special. I eventually found the perfect gown. But three months before the wedding, I started gaining weight. I gained seventeen pounds in three months, just to give you a tiny taste of my dismay. I no longer fit into my wedding gown, and I could not afford to buy another dress two sizes bigger.

I was so confused that I started feeling depressed. My fiancé was beyond mystified. What happened to his carefree, loving, supportive, spontaneous, and fun wife-to-be? Who was this raging, mad woman that "lost it" over the most minor events, and attacked unprovoked? I certainly didn't know. No doubt, the man of my dreams didn't know either.

Something was wrong. I was not the same person. I was not comfortable in my own skin. All I wanted to do was hide in a cave and hope that when I emerged, the nightmare would be over. I was two sizes bigger, cranky, bloated, sleepless, and sweaty. In full panic three months before my wedding--the day I had dreamed about my entire life--I scrambled to find answers. It was countdown time, with no room for error. I needed results and fast! As an executive producer and writer for television, I have a career that demands my becoming an expert on many different topics in a short period of time. Being one of the original executive producers to launch the television network Oxygen Media co-founded by Oprah Winfrey, I was profoundly committed to producing stories about incredible women, such as Gloria Steinem, Ann Richards, Anna Deavere Smith, and Julia-Louis Dreyfus. I had the tools, contacts and passion to find answers.

Desperate, I started reading books, researching the Internet, and speaking to experts. I discovered nothing was changing but me! I was doing everything the menopause books and Internet articles suggested, from dieting to exercising, yet nothing seemed to be working. I searched online and in bookstores for the one book that would explain what was happening to me and show me the way out. I read nearly fifty books, but even though they were loaded with all the medical information I needed to understand menopause, none gave me the solution--the program--that I needed to take back my life. What was a menopausal bride to do? I wanted one-stop shopping. I wanted an ultimate plan. And it was up to me to create it.

Inspired by the wedding planner books I used for my wedding, I decided I really needed a menopause planner to help me keep track of hormones, exercise, and my diet the same way I kept track of caterers, florists and dress fittings. Through extensive research, interviews with medical experts, and trial and error, I developed an eight-step program and menopause planner that really worked. My menopause planner gave me the tools I needed to look and feel better in 12 short weeks, and it will do the same for you.

This book is your survival guide to menopause. It will take the mystery out of menopause, offer you proven solutions to your symptoms, and help you stay sane and organized. With my 12-week program for managing symptoms, you will feel like yourself again in no time!

Thanks to this unusual combination of life transitions--marriage and menopause-- I discovered a wonderful connection: Just as you commit to loving the partner of your dreams, you need to commit to loving yourself. This is especially true during menopause. With The Menopause Makeover, you can say "I do" to the new you.

Before Menopause   During Menopause   After Makeover

MY COMMITMENT TO YOU

The Menopause Makeover produced incredible results, and everyone wanted to know my secret. After my wedding day, I repeated the 12-Week Plan with great success. Knowing that I couldn't be the only one having trouble with menopause, I decided to share what I'd learned to help other women manage menopause. Taking this commitment seriously, I launched a website and crea newsletter to reach out to menopausal women worldwide. The first month, over ten thousand women searching for menopause solutions found the website, women from the U.S.A., Great Britain, Canada, the Bahamas, and Australia. They openly shared their frustrations and concerns. Women wrote to my advice column "Dear Crabby" revealing their deepest fears. I discovered that women were struggling most with weight gain and aging, the very same frustra-tions I was experiencing. Miserable menopause symptoms like hot flashes and dry skin usually came second or third in the list of menopause complaints.

Hearing from other women going through menopause helped me refine the Menopause Makeover program to encompass all of their needs and concerns. The Menopause Makeover of-fers eating and exercise advice, beauty tips, and emotional and relationship support, topped off with a splash of spirituality and a sprinkle of happiness--you need to work on all areas of your life in order to truly manage menopause.

Before publishing this book I spent two years fine-tuning the program, collaborating with medical experts and eventually teaming up with a leading expert on menopause, Dr. Wendy Klein, Associate Professor of Medicine, Obstetrics & Gynecology at Virginia Commonwealth University School of Medicine. As a pioneer in women's health, Dr. Klein shared my passion for helping women manage menopause. We spent months discussing menopause symptoms and treatment solutions, from complementary remedies to hormone therapy, along with the latest scientific evidence on hormone therapy, bioidenticals, and compounded hormones. We read the latest studies from the Women's Health Initiative and leading medical journals on risks associated with hormone therapy, from heart disease to cancer. I was astonished at the misinformation out there in bookstores and online!

Dr. Klein's dedication to accuracy ensures that you have the most up-to-date information at your fingertips. In order to design your own successful Menopause Makeover, you need to be informed and understand all of your choices. In her mission to educate both practitioners and patients, Dr. Klein is committed to healthy solutions based on sound scientific research. I discov-ered that traditional medicine is not only aggressively researching treatment choices for women, but there are already many FDA-approved options available, which are all discussed in this book.

There's a lot of confusion out there about menopause treatment—what's safe, what isn't, what works, and what doesn't. With the help of Dr. Klein, this book provides clear, simple explanations about menopause symptoms and treatment choices. The Menopause Makeover is more than a girlfriend's guide to menopause; it is a book supported by a foundation of sound science. This book is dedicated to your menopausal journey. You have all the tools needed in

The Menopause Makeover to go through "the change" informed with the latest scientific evidence, so you can celebrate your new beginning.

THE MENOPAUSE MAKEOVER IS FOR YOU

When the word *menopause* is used in this book, I am speaking to all women going through perimenopause, menopause, postmenopause and surgical menopause. If you picked up this book, you are suffering from uncomfortable menopausal symptoms and you are looking for:

- Easy-to-understand explanations about what is happening to your ever-changing body and mind
- Treatment options
- New ways of eating and exercising
- Beauty tips that will make you look and feel better

- Solutions to your cranky moods
- Tips that can make sex more enjoyable
- Motivation to accomplish your goals
- A customized plan for surviving—and thriving through--menopause
- Control over your health, your beauty, and your life

Menopause is a natural transition in a woman's life. Yet, it may be the one event that we are least prepared for. From puberty to marriage to new careers to children, each transition is celebrated. We responsibly go through our adult lives taking care of others – our partners, children, family, friends, bosses, co-workers and community – with little left for ourselves. It is understandable that when you reach menopause, it can be overwhelming and confusing. After all, menopause is frustrating! All of a sudden you're dealing with unappealing body changes, uncontrollable crankiness, impatience towards the ones you love, thinning hair, an ever-expanding waistline, difficulty concentrating, and those uninvited hot flashes.

The good news is, it is time to take care of you. Menopause is a time for personal growth, lifestyle changes and new solutions. Unfortunately, nobody gave us a map to navigate this journey in life. You may feel completely out of control, but you can create balance and find joy in the new vibrant you. This book will offer you individual options – from hormone choices to eating and exercise plans. Because we all experience menopause differently, you must create a plan that fits your needs.

You are not alone. By the year 2020, the number of U.S. women older than 51 (the average age menopause can occur naturally), is expected to be more than 50 million. According to the North American Menopause Society, every day an estimated six thousand women have reached menopause in North America - that's over 2 million per year! Currently, over 20 percent of our female baby boomers are slamming into one of the stages of menopause. Approximately 80 percent of these women will experience uncomfortable symptoms such as hot flashes, weight gain, fuzzy thinking, and low sex drive that can lead to irritability. You are not losing your mind. Rather, you are gaining an opportunity to create new beginnings!

Whether your menopause symptoms are mild or severe, this planner will help you feel better and take charge of your health. Menopause is more than fluctuating hormones and hot flashes; it is also a time to look at your life. It is the beginning of a new chapter and an opportunity for self-renewal. Are you happy? Is it time for a tune-up? Or a major overhaul? It was for me.

I made a number of startling discoveries during my 12-Week Menopause Makeover – some exciting, some discouraging. It became clear that I needed to exercise five to six days a week to be healthy. I had to eat more protein and fewer pastries, and cut my portions. My skincare routine had to be modified. My unhealthy relationships had to be addressed. I had to create a partnership with my doctor. And my self-image had to be readjusted. I had to get comfortable in my new skin.

Transitions can be scary and exciting; it is how we look at the journey that makes the difference. Planning a wedding can be stressful, yet it is also joyful, a time of celebration. Why can't the menopausal transition, complete with undesirable symptoms wrapped with midlife changes, be an exciting time, a time of celebration too? A new beginning? If we throw parties for Sweet 16, graduation, bridal showers, and baby showers, we should throw hot flash parties, too!

HOW TO USE THIS BOOK

When you are planning a wedding, there is a clear-cut agenda and timeline, a team to help you, and a list of choices to make and questions to answer. No two weddings are alike; it's up to you to design the wedding of your dreams. This book utilizes a similar step-by-step strategy, incorporating tips, checklists, and calendars to help you design a personal action plan—a menopause makeover designed by you, for you.

THE THREE PART PROGRAM

The Menopause Makeover is an easy-to-use three-part process.

PART ONE: "Your Menopause Survival Guide" is the powerful 8-step program. These 8 steps are the actual makeover—your physical, emotional, and spiritual program to look and feel better. Each chapter in Part One will give you the information you need to be successful, complete with help-ful charts and checklists.

PART TWO: "Your Menopause Makeover: Planning your Transformation" gives you the tools to customize your makeover. In Part Two, you'll take stock of where you are today and set personal goals for your 12-Week Makeover.

PART THREE: "Your Menopause Makeover Essential Planner: Twelve Weeks to a New You" provides you with all the tools you need to achieve your makeover goals. Part three is your essential planner. It includes the forms you need to keep on track, self-assessments to chart your progress, and delicious recipes to feed the new you. Documenting your journey can be rewarding especially when you start to see the results.

After I said, "I do" to this Menopause Makeover plan, I never looked back. When I started on this journey, I had a long way to go. I had to learn to love the new me. I had to learn to be grateful for what I had. I had to learn to be compassionate towards myself, yet determined to make changes. I had to admit I was starting to age (gulp), and that was a biggie. Today, I feel more vibrant and sexier than ever before. It took hard work, but with this 12-Week, 8-step program I was able to see the areas where I was failing, and the areas that were working well.

If you're struggling through menopause like I was, and want to feel better, look better, and be healthy, then The Menopause Makeover is for you. If you do the work, you will see the results. Trust me—if I could do it, you can, too!

QUIZ |Are you ready for a *Menopause Makeover?*	Yes	No
1. Have you gained more than ten pounds in the past year?	✓	
2. Have you tried other diets without success?	✓	
3. Are you perimenopausal, menopausal, postmenopausal?	✓	
4. Experiencing menopausal symptoms, such as hot flashes?	✓	
5. Have you lost your waistline?	✓	
6. Do you make excuses for not wanting to have sex?	✓	
7. Do you have cravings for sugar, salt, or alcohol?	✓	
8. Are you hungry all the time?	✓	
9. Are you not seeing results like you used to from exercise?	✓	
10. Are you depressed?	✓	
11. Are you buying bigger clothes this year?	✓	
12. Are you between the ages 38-58?	✓	
13. Do you feel like the "normal" you is a thing of the past?	✓	
14. Are you cranky and irritable?	✓	
15. Do you have less patience for loved ones?	✓	

If you answered, "yes" to at least 10 of the above questions, it is time to regain control of your health and beauty again. It is time to start *The Menopause Makeover!*

PART 1

Your Menopause Survival Guide: Eight Steps to a Complete Makeover

Chapter 1	Wait a Minute…What Just Happened? Your Body During Menopause

Feeling blue, gaining weight, suffering from hot flashes, being cranky, losing interest in sex, and forgetting things – this had become my new daily reality. If that were not enough, I had to start slapping on gallons of facial moisturizer, hoping my once radiant complexion would return.

Feeling helpless, frustrated and desperate for a solution, I scheduled an appointment to see my doctor. After the examination and a tearful discussion including my confession-- "I think I am losing my mind" --the doctor gave me an FSH blood test. Praying I didn't have a strange disease causing all this misery, I eagerly awaited the results.

A week later, the doctor phoned, "I have good news. You're not losing your mind. You don't have a disease. You're going through menopause." I said, "What! I'm *what*? Not me? Wait a minute…what just happened?"

Shocked, standing there with the phone in my hand, I felt that life as I knew it was over. Menopause had never even occurred to me; I was totally blindsided. Surely this was not happening to *me*. My favorite blouse was suddenly drenched from an uninvited hot flash. My mind was fuzzy as I tried to focus on the clock pounding over the kitchen sink--*tick, tock, tick, tock*--or was that my heart? It certainly wasn't my egg count--that was now *tocked*!

I was scared – something I took for granted had just been taken away without my permission. The sunlight was streaming through the kitchen window, giving me a glimmer of hope that there must be a way to make this go away. I took a deep breath, and said, "OK, give me something to fix this."

Well, the hard truth is there is no magic pill that will "fix" menopause. Believe me, I tried to find one. The good news is you can manage menopause. The first step is to understand your symptoms and your treatment options. If you know your options, you can manage menopause.

You may be feeling miserable and frustrated, wanting to feel "normal" again-- and fast. Fortunately, you have a big advantage in your life you may not be acknowledging--unlike other transitions, now you have a lifetime of experience at hand! You are already equipped with survival tools and coping skills. You managed to make it through puberty, perhaps marriage, divorce, children, financial challenges, family issues, and career ups and downs. If you have gotten this far in life, hot flashes, a few new wrinkles, a declining libido and weight gain are all conditions you can manage. You are armed with a lifetime of knowledge. Once you make up your mind to meet these issues head-on, you are ready to walk through a new door and realize your new powerful potential!

WHAT IS MENOPAUSE?

As I urgently searched for answers to my severe menopause symptoms and cranky moods, it occurred to me that this was a time in my life that demanded attention. The word *menopause* took on a new meaning for me: ME-NO-PAUSE. I could no longer give all of my attention to others. I now had to focus on "ME." I could "NO" longer "PAUSE" on matters regarding "ME."

Menopause is actually derived from the Greek roots *meno* (month) and *pausis* (a pause, a cessation). Menopause, the natural stopping of your reproductive cycle, is a completely normal physical transition in a woman's life. The dictionary defines *menopause* as "the time in a woman's life when menstruation diminishes and ceases, usually between the ages of 45 and 55."

The menopause journey has three stages. Perimenopause (*peri* is Latin meaning "around" or "near") is the time prior to the cessation of menstruation, when you begin to experience hormonal changes and you are still having intermittent periods. Many doctors now refer to perimenopause as the menopausal transition. I will refer to it this way as well. You have reached menopause once you have gone 12 months without a period. Postmenopause is the time after menopause when the acute symptoms of estrogen absence generally diminish.

Going through the menopausal transition is the reverse of puberty. Puberty was the transition in your life when your hormones were gearing up for the reproductive years. Remember your first period? Emotional outbursts, tender breasts, restless nights, and feeling bloated?

THREE STAGES OF MENOPAUSE

PERIMENOPAUSE: The phase leading up to menopause when your hormones start changing. In this stage, you may experience symptoms such as hot flashes and irregular periods. This transition can last up to six years.

MENOPAUSE: Once you have gone 12 months without a period, you are considered to be in menopause.

POSTMENOPAUSE: The years after you've reached menopause.

YOUR HORMONES DURING MENOPAUSE

During the transition into menopause, you may experience many of the same puberty symptoms, but for different reasons. Instead of turning on your hormones, your body is now turning them off by slowly producing less estrogen and progesterone.

THE LEADING LADY AND COSTARS OF MENOPAUSE

Estrogen is the feminizing hormone responsible for maintaining the health of reproductive tissue, breasts, skin and brain. Estrogen is secreted mostly from the ovaries. We make three types of estrogen:

Estradiol – The dominant, most biologically active estrogen produced by the ovaries before menopause.

Estrone – The most abundant estrogen made by your body after menopause: less potent than estradiol. Before menopause it was produced by your ovaries but was inactive.

Estriol – Increases during pregnancy: less potent than estradiol.

Progesterone is a hormone produced by the ovaries and by the placenta. Progesterone helps prepares the uterus for pregnancy. When you are pregnant, progesterone also stimulates the mammary glands and maintains the pregnancy.

Testosterone, another hormone secreted from the ovaries and adrenal glands, started slowing down before menopause. It influences your energy and libido. Men generate over 20 times more testosterone than women. The ovaries and adrenal glands produce testosterone. After menopause we produce about half the amount of testosterone.

Follicle-stimulating hormone (FSH) is secreted by the pituitary gland, and triggers the growth of eggs in the ovaries and estrogen production starting the ovulation cycle.

Luteinizing hormone (LH) is secreted by the pituitary gland and stimulates ovulation.

Many women who had severe symptoms during puberty may also have a challenging menopause while women who slid through adolescence easily often have the same experience with menopause. We are all different and menopause is no exception. In order to fully understand menopause, we must look at how our bodies have been operating since birth.

We are born with a finite number of eggs, about 1 to 2 million, stored in small follicles in our ovaries. From birth to puberty, the majority of eggs will die. At puberty, about 400,000 remain. Each month in which we have a period, about 1,000 eggs are lost and usually only one actually matures into a fertile egg (ovum). A woman will have about 500 ovulations.

The ovaries not only hold these eggs, but also produce the hormones estrogen and progesterone. During days 1 to 14 of your cycle, a hormone called follicle-stimulating hormone (FSH) is produced by your pituitary gland in the brain. It stimulates the growth of immature follicles to maturation and to make estrogen. Once there is a sufficient level of estrogen in your body, usually around day twelve to sixteen of your cycle, the pituitary gland sends luteinizing hormone (LH) to signal the follicle to release the egg (ovulation).

Once ovulation has occurred, your estrogen levels drop and progesterone starts to rise. By day twenty, progesterone levels are high enough to prepare the uterus for pregnancy. If the egg is fertilized, your progesterone levels will remain high. If the egg is not fertilized, both estrogen and progesterone levels fall and you start your period. This process is called the menstrual cycle. During menopause your body begins to produce less estrogen and progesterone causing this cycle to become irregular, and eventually ending.

WHY DOES MENOPAUSE OCCUR?

Since you're born with a finite number of eggs, the number of follicles in your ovaries decreases over time. The ovaries also start to produce lower levels of hormones. Menopause occurs when the ovaries stop making enough hormones to stimulate your monthly cycle.

SO HOW DO I KNOW IT'S MENOPAUSE?

As your hormones start changing and your body enters the menopausal transition, there are a number of factors that will help confirm whether you are experiencing symptoms associated with perimenopause or menopause. If you think you are experiencing one of the stages of menopause, visit your doctor or health practitioner. This is a perfect time to reassess your health and to be proactive about preventive measures and health screening.

Communicating with your clinician is important. You need to give her all the information she needs to make an accurate evaluation. Next you will review different treatment options. It will take a joint effort with your practitioner to successfully diagnosis and manage your menopause. If your symptoms are not being properly treated, seek a second opinion. The North American Menopause Society has a resource that lists knowledgeable doctors belonging to their organization. (See the Author's Note at the back of the book.)

MAKING THE MOST OF YOUR DOCTOR'S VISIT

Be prepared! Here are helpful tips on how to provide your practitioner with the information she needs to make an accurate diagnosis and evaluate your symptoms making the most out of your visit.

Before Your Appointment:

- List your current symptoms and their severity level.
- Note your menstrual patterns.
- List all recent medical issues and physical concerns.
- List your personal medical history.
- List your family medical history.
- Make a list of all medications and vitamins you are currently taking.
- Think about treatment choices ahead of time and come prepared with questions to ask.

After Your Physical Examination:

- Ask if your personal or family medical history will influence your treatment choices.
- Discuss having a follicle stimulating hormone (FSH) blood test.
- Discuss other medical testing you may need at this stage of your life, such as mammograms, bone density testing, colonoscopy, and lipid profiles.

After you discuss your medical history, testing, treatment options and current medications, and you decide on a course of action, make sure to ask your doctor about side effects, benefits, risks, and length of treatment. Also discuss your risk of postmenopausal osteoporosis and whether you still need to practice birth control.

For helpful forms to prepare for your appointment, see Chapter 13, "The Essential Planner."

In order to make the most of your doctor's visit, it's helpful to come prepared.

Bring the list of suggested information from "Making the Most of Your Doctor's Visit" to your next appointment. This information will help facilitate your conversation and result in a more thorough evaluation. Menopause can be a complex transition. The more information your practitioner has the better the odds of properly managing your menopause symptoms.

It is important that you trust your health practitioner and feel comfortable discussing anything from sex to hot flashes. A good relationship will be rewarding in the long run!

MENOPAUSE TESTS

Your practitioner may decide to give you a blood test to determine where you are in the menopause process. There are a number of different tests available. The most reliable test is the follicle-stimulating hormone blood test.

FSH (FOLLICLE-STIMULATING HORMONE) BLOOD LEVEL TEST

The FSH (follicle-stimulating hormone) blood level test is a simple blood sample that can be taken at your doctor's office or a lab. As the number of follicles decline over the years, your FSH levels rise. If you still get your period, you should have this test on the third to fifth day of your period. If you no longer get a period, you can take this test at any time. Since hormone levels fluctuate, it is often a good idea to repeat this blood test in one to three months to confirm the results.

The FSH blood test is generally a good indicator as to where you are in the menopause transition. A higher number indicates that you are closer to menopause. When your FSH is elevated, it is a sign that your pituitary is working hard to stimulate ovulation, even when the ovaries are no longer able to ovulate in response.

WHAT DO THE RESULTS MEAN?

PERIMENOPAUSE: Levels above 25 mIU/mL (milli-international units per milliliter) likely signal that the ovaries are just starting to cease estrogen production.

MENOPAUSE: FSH levels 40 or above generally indicate that your ovaries aren't producing enough estrogen to maintain your monthly cycle. You may still get your periods intermittently even though your ovaries have started to decrease their hormonal activity.

POSTMENOPAUSE: Levels 40 to 135.

There is some variability among laboratories – your clinician will be able to interpret the results.

HORMONE BLOOD LEVEL TESTS

Many doctors test individual hormones, such as estradiol or testosterone. Hormones vary significantly from day to day, and from individual to individual, so these are not generally useful tests when treating menopause symptoms, as your hormone levels often won't correspond to symptoms.

URINE AND SALIVA HOME TESTS

There are also urine and saliva tests you can do at home to check your FSH and hormone levels. Although popular, these tests are not as accurate as the FSH blood test, and there is no sound scientific evidence to guide their use.

Because your body and hormones are changing daily, a simple FSH blood test may be a useful step to a correct diagnosis. That being said, no one test can accurately evaluate your menopause status. Your body is constantly changing, and your symptoms may change. To properly "test" for menopause, your practitioner should review your overall health profile.

UNDERSTANDING YOUR MENOPAUSE SYMPTOMS

Once you establish that you are in one of the stages of menopause, understanding your symptoms is the first step to managing them. Your symptoms can give you clues as to what your body is experiencing. This will help when deciding what course of action to pursue. Some women will experience very troubling symptoms, while others slide through the menopause transition without a hot flash. How you experience and manage your transition will be unique to you. We are all different!

Tracking your symptoms may be the most useful information used in treating menopause. Your body is giving you clues that you can use to restore balance. Just as a detective collects evidence to solve a case, you too can collect information and solve *your* case. Your symptoms will guide you throughout your menopausal journey as they continue to change until postmenopause. We all know that experiencing menopause symptoms can be challenging, but it can be fascinating to witness your body's sophisticated orchestration between you and your hormones.

Compare the complex mechanisms in a watch to the effects hormones have on our body. A watch has many interlocking gears. One turns the other. Some are big and some are small. When one does not function properly, it causes a cascading affect on the others. Similarly, the interplay of reproductive hormones is extremely complex; they affect one another. Often your symptoms will tell you what "gear" is out-of-whack, so you can consider the best approach.

Document your symptoms using this checklist before starting your Menopause Makeover. Revisit this checklist in three months after completing the 12-Week Plan. Are your symptoms better? Worse? Do you have new symptoms? Many symptoms experienced during the menopausal transition are hormone-related, but many are age-related. Once you document your current menopause symptom status, use this information to discuss treatment options with your healthcare provider. If your symptoms are mild and tolerable, they are likely to resolve without any treatment at all.

Symptoms Checklist

Do you experience any of these symptoms? If so, check off the symptoms that apply to you and rate the level of intensity with 1 being mild and 10 being miserable, then record the date. Use this checklist to discuss your symptoms with your doctor.

Physical signs	Intensity (1-10)	Date	Psychological signs	Intensity (1-10)	Date
Irregular periods			Mood swings		
Hot flashes			Crankiness		
Night sweats			Memory loss		
Weight gain			Sleep problems		
Breast tenderness			Loss of libido		
Heart palpitations			Depression		
Migraine headaches			Fatigue		
Bladder changes			Anxiety		
Incontinence					
Vaginal dryness					
Vision changes					
Joint aches					
Muscle tension					
Teeth and gum problems					
Skin changes					
Hair changes					
Fluid retention and bloating					
Increased blood pressure					

WHAT MENOPAUSAL SYMPTOMS ARE YOU EXPERIENCING?

Many of the symptoms you're experiencing are very common for menopausal women. You're not alone! The following lists the causes and solutions for the most common symptoms—go through it and note which symptoms you've been experiencing. Speak to your practitioner about the approach that might be right for you.

IRREGULAR PERIODS

This is probably the first symptom that you noticed. When you first start to go through menopause, your periods start to get a bit unpredictable. You may notice spotting, heavier or lighter bleeding and your periods may be longer or shorter.

CAUSES: When the ovaries run out of functioning eggs and hormone secretion is erratic, your natural cycle changes. Some months you may ovulate and some months you may not.

SOLUTIONS: Keep track of your periods in the Essential Planner. What date does your period start? How long does it last? Is bleeding heavy or light? Are you suffering from cramps? When appropriate, a low dose of birth control pills can regulate your periods, with the added benefit of birth control.

HOT FLASHES

The most common and most irritating symptom associated with menopause is hot flashes. Up to 80 percent of women going through menopause experience hot flashes. A hot flash is a feeling of warmth to intense heat on the upper body and face lasting 1 to 5 minutes, sometimes followed by chills. Your heart rate can also increase, up to 7 to 15 beats more per minute.

CAUSES: Those ever-changing hormones cause hot flashes. When estrogen levels fall, your body's thermostat, located in the brain (hypothalamus), may have a hard time regulating your body temperature. Some women are more sensitive than others to this temperature change. We are all different, so frequency, duration and intensity may vary. The good news is hot flashes usually decline two years after postmenopause, although some women have them longer.

There are also non-hormonal causes for hot flashes. Being overweight, smoking, suffering from diabetes, infection, malignancies, autoimmune disorders, under- or over-active thyroid, some medications, such as SERMs or SSRIs can also cause hot flashes. Yet, even the healthiest person living a stress-free lifestyle can experience hot flashes. There is nothing fun about hot flashes. They usually come on at the most inconvenient times.

SOLUTIONS: There is hope! Start documenting the times you suffer from hot flashes in your daily planner. Are they triggered by alcohol? Spicy foods? Caffeine? Heat? Smoking cigarettes? Are you asleep? Are you under stress? Determine your hot flash triggers and avoid them. Wear layered clothing. Sip a cool beverage. Sit near the air conditioner. Carry a cute hand fan. Being prepared is your first course of action. Often low-dose hormone therapy (HT) can bring hot flash relief. Other medications, including antidepressants, anti-seizure drugs, and some herbs may also be helpful in relieving hot flashes. Enjoy a yoga class, schedule a massage or relaxing bath. Regular exercise is a must, and you should maintain a healthy weight. If you smoke, stop! Review your medications with your clinician and make sure they are not causing hot flashes.

NIGHT SWEATS

When you're sleeping, it is normal for your body temperature to drop slightly. However, thrashing around in bed all night from uncomfortable nighttime sweating followed by a cold sensation can be a drag and promise a day of irritability.

CAUSES: Low or fluctuating hormone levels can disturb the body's thermostat for many.

If you wake up sweating, that cooling system in your brain is stimulating the sweat glands.

SOLUTIONS: Sleep in cotton PJ's on cotton sheets. Set up an electric fan next to your side of the bed, and lower your thermostat before going to bed. Avoid caffeine drinks, no alcohol or nicotine close to bedtime. Sleep at regular hours. Make sure your bedroom is dark and keep the temperature cool. Exercise daily, but not within three hours of bedtime. If you are experiencing stress, meditate and relax.

WEIGHT GAIN

One of the most frustrating symptom during menopause, is weight gain. The average woman gains one pound per year starting around the age of 40, thanks to aging and a lower metabolism.

CAUSES: Only some weight gain can be blamed on our changing hormones. Over the years, many of us have had less time to exercise and eat properly, and when we enter menopause the effects are unforgiving. During menopause, it is natural for the body to store fat around your "middle," so that your waistline starts to disappear. It is often typical to gain 5 to 10 pounds during menopause transition, but more than that suggests the need to make changes in your lifestyle!

SOLUTIONS: A commitment to healthy food choices and daily exercise is a vital step toward feeling better and taking control of your health. *Menopausal weight gain is a wake-up call.* Set weight goals and track your weight for the next 12 weeks in the Essential Planner. More information and solutions to weight gain in Chapter 3.

BREAST TENDERNESS

Breast tissue is sensitive to hormonal change and can sometimes feel tender. Many women notice tender breasts when they first begin hormone therapy.

CAUSES: Hormonal changes may cause fluid retention in your breasts, similar to your monthly cycle experience. Once your hormones are stabilized, you will notice this uncomfortable symptom subsiding.

SOLUTIONS: Cut back on your caffeine and salt consumption.

HEART PALPITATIONS

Have you ever felt like your heart was pounding out of your chest? During menopause, heart palpitations can be scary, and can happen at inappropriate times. Sometimes palpitations accompany hot flashes. This double whammy is no fun!

Causes: No one knows for sure why some women suffer from heart palpitations during menopause. It is often attributed to hormonal fluctuation.

Solutions: If you suspect heart disease or if heart disease runs in your family, be sure to discuss these symptoms with your health-care provider.

MIGRAINE HEADACHES

If migraine headaches are new to you, or if they only happened during the first few days of your period or during ovulation, you may be responding to changing estrogen levels. Do you have triggers? Alcohol? Spicy food? Temperature change? Stress? Dieting? Caffeine? Certain foods? Medications? Are you suffering from a sinus infection, dental issues, or allergies? There is hope that migraines that appear during menopause will often subside during postmenopause.

Causes: There have been studies that established a connection between migraines and menstrual periods for some women. During perimenopause, fluctuating estrogen levels may trigger more migraines than you experienced during a normal cycle.

Solutions: Leveling hormones alleviates migraines for some women, but for others, hormone therapy makes the headaches worse. If you have tension headaches nonprescription medications, such as aspirin, or anti-inflammatory medications (such as ibuprofen) can offer relief. Do you have triggers? Alcohol? Spicy food? Stress? Practice stress management and relaxation techniques. Small studies have suggested riboflavin, magnesium and/or coenzyme Q10 are nonprescription medications that may help reduce your migraines, if taken daily. Prescription medicines are available to help with migraines. Speak to your clinician about your options.

BLADDER CHANGES/INCONTINENCE

There is nothing worse than hurrying to find a bathroom when you've gotta go. Up to 60 percent of all women 45 to 55 years of age suffer from mild incontinence, so you are not alone.

Causes: Common culprits are age, obesity, family history, childbearing trauma, hysterectomy and smoking/chronic coughing.

Solutions: Before visiting your healthcare provider, keep a 3-day diary recording how many times a day you urinate, whether it wakes you up at night, whether urine leaks out before you get to the bathroom or the front door, or when you sneeze or cough. Also record your fluid intake. Wear a light minipad; it is much easier to change than your panties or slacks. Make sure you pee after every meal. Treatments for incontinence include Kegel exercises, avoiding bladder irritants (caffeine, soda, tomatoes, grapefruit juice), fluid restrictions, bladder training, and urination at timed intervals.

VAGINAL DRYNESS

Vaginal dryness is not only a common menopause symptom, it can actually affect your sexual desire and pleasure. With dryness, your vagina can become irritated more easily from friction, and the vaginal tissues may lose their elasticity.

CAUSES: When your estrogen levels drop, vaginal dryness can occur. Estrogen plumps up the cells in the vaginal wall so they produce more lubrication.

SOLUTIONS: For a quick fix, try a bioadhesive lubricant, such as AstroGlide or vaginal moisturizer, such as Replens. Estrogen improves lubrication, keeping vaginal tissues working properly. Low-dose hormone therapy or estrogen creams applied vaginally, may alleviate vaginal dryness. If you suffer from a number of menopause symptoms, oral hormone therapy may be a better option. More information, see Chapter 7.

SKIN CHANGES

No one escapes the aging process. Sun damage, smoking, eating poorly and inadequate skincare are big contributors to sagging and wrinkling skin. For those of you who loved getting a summer suntan, the effects of sun on your skin are damaging. Gravity takes its toll on everyone who has spent 40-plus years on this planet, but what most of us notice during menopause is that the elasticity and firmness of our skin decreases.

CAUSES: The skin is supported by collagen and elastin fibers, which are supported by estrogen.

Hormone changes can affect the skin's physiology, with almost 30percent of the skin's collagen depleted the first five years after menopause.

SOLUTIONS: Wear sunscreen with a sun protection factor (SPF) 15+ daily--this is not negotiable if you want healthy skin. Antioxidants and topical retinoids can help sun damaged skin. Exfoliate regularly, and moisturize daily. This is a perfect time for a new skin regime. For more skincare information, including non-surgical cosmetic treatments, see Chapter 5.

HAIR CHANGES

During menopause 40 to 50 percent of women report some hair loss or thinning, called androgenic alopecia (AGA). Perhaps, you are sprouting facial hair? Is it coarse? Does it appear on the chin, upper lip and cheeks? Then you may be one of the 5 to 15 percent of women who experience hirsutism (presence of excess hair). Some women experience excessive peach fuzz or discover rogue hairs.

CAUSES: Having too much or too little hair during midlife can be caused by changing hormones, age, genetics, metabolism, high blood pressure medication, depression, thyroid disease, chemotherapy, or stress. Androgenic alopecia (AGA) or hair thinning is often genetic. Did your mom or dad have thinning hair?

SOLUTIONS: To treat hair thinning, try topical minoxidil solution (Rogaine 2%). It is the only over-the-counter drug available to promote hair growth in women with androgenic alopecia.

If you only have a few rogue hairs try tweezing, shaving, depilatory hair creams, or waxing. Dark peach fuzz can often be treated with facial bleach products or waxing. Electrolysis is another option. Vaniqa cream (not available in Canada) is a prescription topical enzyme inhibitor of hair growth. More information, see Chapter 5.

FLUID RETENTION & BLOATING

Remember feeling bloated during your period? If a few days a month weren't bad enough, when you go through the menopausal transition, this can persist for months on end!

CAUSES: The causes of bloating vary. Irregular ovarian function and fluctuating estrogen levels during menopause can cause bloating. Poor nutrition and high salt intake can also cause bloating.

SOLUTIONS: In the Essential Planner, note the days you feel bloated and decrease your salt intake these days. A high-potassium diet may help provide bloating relief. High potassium foods include all meats, poultry and fish, apricots, avocado, banana, cantaloupe, kiwi, lima beans, milk, oranges, potatoes, prunes, spinach, tomatoes, and winter squash.

MOOD SWINGS AND CRANKINESS

Are you experiencing a lot of change and stress lately? Midlife stressors such as relationship issues, losses, caring for parents, or career issues can make you moody.

CAUSES: Hormonal flux can make the best of us moody and cranky. Throw in hot flashes, weight gain, and a dry vagina-- no wonder you are moody and cranky!

SOLUTIONS: If you are experiencing mood swings, this is a good time in your life to start making time to relax, meditate, take yoga, enjoy herbal teas, and pamper yourself. Exercise and good nutrition will help. For more information, see Chapter 6.

MEMORY LOSS

Forget your car keys? Forget an appointment? Repeat the same thing a few times only to be corrected by your listener? Short-term memory loss or fuzzy thinking is common during menopause.

CAUSES: The effects of estrogen, age, stress, medications and overall health can affect your memory. Fluctuating hormones can mess with the connections in your brain, short-circuiting your memory. Night sweats, lack of sleep, midlife stress and hot flashes can contribute to memory loss.

SOLUTIONS: Ask your loved ones for support. Get organized with planners and calendars. Keep your mind active, and enjoy a healthy lifestyle. Make sure you get good night's sleep. A rested mind can absorb more information. Find out more, see Chapter 6.

SLEEP PROBLEMS

If you are experiencing night sweats, it is no surprise you are not sleeping at night. A sleepless night will promise a day of irritability and mood swings. Nonmenopausal sleep problems can also contribute to sleepless nights. Consuming food, caffeine, or alcohol just before bedtime, and bad habits like watching TV in bed can keep you awake.

CAUSES: Anxiety, mood swings, hot flashes, itchy skin, and suffering from depression can all contribute to sleepless nights.

SOLUTIONS: Avoid stimulants such as exercise and caffeine in the evening, and no excessive day-time napping. If your sleepless nights are caused by menopause symptoms, a low-dose hormone therapy may bring back restful sleep. Prescription sleep aids are another option. Discuss with your healthcare provider. Keep a "sleep diary" in your 12-Week Planner under "Notes." Track the time you fell asleep, the time you woke up, what you ate before sleeping, and how many times you woke up during the night.

LOSS OF LIBIDO

Not feeling sexy? Between the ages of 55 and 65, sexual desire may diminish for men and women. Once we exit the reproducing stage of our life, we may experience a loss of libido.

CAUSES: Aging, along with changing hormone levels, may blow the flame of desire out of your love life. Declining levels of estrogen and testosterone may also contribute to decreased libido. Suffering from menopause symptoms including vaginal dryness may squash any interest in sex. Refer to "vaginal dryness" in Chapter 7. Physical, emotional and social factors can all affect your libido. Certain medications for blood pressure, depression, heart disease, or diabetes can decrease your libido as well.

SOLUTIONS: Discuss your declining libido with your practitioner. If you need to treat the relationship, seek counseling. Schedule romantic dates with your loved one, exercise to increase your "feel good" hormones, enjoy an alcoholic beverage to loosen up (in moderation), try new routines in bed with your partner. A healthy and active sex life is possible during and after menopause. See Chapter 7 for more information

DEPRESSION

If you are suffering from hopelessness, apprehension, and deep sadness for prolonged periods (two weeks or longer) you may be depressed. Do you feel worthless? Have you lost interest in your favorite activities? Are you angry? Have you felt hopeless? If you are suffering from lifestyle stress (change in relationship, finances, loss of a loved one, caring for parents) seek support.

CAUSES: Depression is an illness that can be triggered by the chemicals in your brain. Serotonin regulates your moods. It is the "feel good" hormone. When serotonin levels drop due to fluctuating hormones, you can experience extreme episodes of depression. Some medications can worsen depression. It is important to review your medications with your practitioner.

SOLUTIONS: There is hope – hormone therapy, antidepressants and psychotherapy can help you if you are suffering from depression. If you have a history of suffering from clinical depression, be sure to discuss with your practitioner. For more information, see Chapter 6.

ANXIETY

Feeling wound up, like you may explode at any minute? Mild intermittent anxiety sometimes occurs during the menopausal transition. Generally these symptoms will subside over time. **CAUSES:** Going through physical, emotional, and midlife lifestyle changes can cause anxiety.

Solutions: Discuss your anxiety with your loved ones and friends; support can make a difference during anxiety attacks. If your anxiety seems out of control, discuss with your health-care provider.

Once you understand your body's changes, it will be easier to manage menopause. Identifying your personal symptoms is the first step in creating a plan that fits your lifestyle.

Now that you know about menopause, why it happens, the stages, and how it affects your life, you may be asking, "What do I do about it?" This is where the fun begins. *The Menopause Makeover* has an 8-Step, 12-Week program that will give you the tools to do something about "it!"

| Chapter 2 | Step One: OK, So I'm Menopausal… Now What Do I Do? Understanding Your Treatment Options |

Once you know that you are perimenopausal or menopausal, you're probably wondering, "So, what can I do to feel better? " With numerous medical studies on hormone therapy, and an abundance of purported remedies, making the correct choice can be difficult.

When I stopped taking birth control pills, I slammed into menopause riddled with severe symptoms. I tried doing nothing, hoping I could tolerate these menopausal changes, but without success. Then I opted for some popular herbal remedies, whose properties for overcoming menopausal symptoms I know are scientifically unfounded. Not surprisingly, I had no success. Next, I attempted visualization exercises hoping that "seeing" a life free of hot flashes would help. That did not work. I even prayed nightly, asking God to "please relieve my hot flashes!" God was listening, because I finally got it right. By combining hormone therapy (HT), complementary remedies (yoga and carefully selected supplements), as well as developing new exercise routines, and committing to a new eating plan, I started feeling better. It took a combination of treatment options to regain control of my health and well-being. It took hard work. The payoff was the renewal of a happy and healthy me.

We are all different. No two of us have the same history, genetics, beliefs, or comfort zones. Because there is no one formula, no magic pill, it can be challenging to treat menopause symptoms. If you have a family history of osteoporosis, heart disease or cancer, your treatment choices are critical to your health. It is important that you take an active interest in managing your menopause, incorporating your personal beliefs, your genetic history, and your current medical concerns. Because we have choices, we can find solutions.

The first step to creating a menopause management plan is to understand your treatment options.

OPTIONS FOR TREATING MENOPAUSE

- Lifestyle changes, such as diet and exercise
- Hormone therapy
- Complementary And Alternative (CAM) practices
- A combination of the above

LIFESTYLE CHANGES

Studies have clearly shown that good lifestyle habits, such as proper nutrition and regular exercise, can benefit your overall health. Being committed to good health, including no smoking and limited alcohol consumption, will give you more energy and help you sleep better. In addition, your mood and general outlook often improve. While there have been no formal studies that confirm diet and exercise alleviate menopausal symptoms, I can confirm that I felt better after I lost weight and incorporated exercise into my daily routine. My high blood pressure went down and I enjoyed shopping for new clothes as a reward for my victories. Practicing healthy lifestyle habits is important during this phase of your life. The habits you establish now could add years to your life. There is more information about nutrition in Chapter 3 and about exercise in Chapter 4.

HORMONE THERAPY

If you have severe menopausal symptoms, you may be a good candidate for hormone therapy. Hormone therapy (HT) is used to supplement the body with estrogen when the ovaries no longer produce adequate levels and can help alleviate many of your symptoms, including hot flashes, vaginal dryness, and night sweats. In 2012 a new study, KEEPS, concluded that estrogen/progesterone treatment started soon after menopause appears to be safe; relieves many of the symptoms of menopause; and improves mood, bone density, and several markers of cardiovascular risk.

Since estrogen alone has been found to increase the risk of uterine cancer, most HT consists of progesterone along with estrogen, which eliminates that cancer risk. If a woman has had a hysterectomy, and thus does not have a uterus, she does not need to take progesterone and can take estrogen by itself.

While hormone therapy can reduce the risk of some disorders or diseases (colon cancer, osteoporosis, vaginal atrophy), it can also increase the risk of others such as breast cancer and blood clots. If you are at risk for breast cancer, blood clots or uterine (endometrial) cancer, discuss these issues with your doctor before starting hormone therapy.

Hormone therapy may seem intimidating at first, but it's really not that complicated—all you need to do is understand your options to decide what's right for you. At first, when discussing hormone therapy with my doctor, I was intrigued by transdermal application and bioidenticals. After trying this choice, I found I did not actually like wearing a patch or applying creams. I preferred taking a pill, and I was a good candidate, so I take a pill every morning. Once you learn the basics, you will be able to discuss your preferences with your healthcare provider. Let's get started!

WHAT TYPE OF HORMONE THERAPY IS RIGHT FOR YOU?

All women are different. Your medical history and genetics make you unique. Treating menopause symptoms and long-term health is very personal to each woman. When discussing hormone therapy (HT), there are two basic options: estrogen therapy (ET) and estrogen plus progestogen therapy (EPT). The term hormone therapy (HT) covers both ET and EPT. The FDA refers to EPT as HT.

HORMONE THERAPY TERMINOLOGY

ESTROGEN THERAPY (ET): Estrogen alone, or "unopposed" estrogen, is prescribed for postmenopausal women who have had a hysterectomy. This is because without a uterus, the risk of uterine cancer is essentially absent, so there is no need for the uterine protection of progesterone.

ESTROGEN PLUS PROGESTOGEN THERAPY (EPT): A combination of both estrogen and progestogen (either progesterone or progestin, synthetic forms of progesterone). Progesterone coupled with estrogen eliminates the risk of uterine cancer, by preventing stimulation of the uterine lining.

WAYS TO TAKE HORMONE THERAPY

Hormone therapy can be administered vaginally (with vaginal creams, rings or suppositories), through the bloodstream (pills) or transdermally (through the skin).

WAYS HORMONE THERAPY CAN BE ADMINISTERED

- Oral – the most commonly used formulation
- Transdermal – patch, gel, and spray
- Vaginal – creams, rings and tablets
- Intrauterine Device (IUD) – progesterone only

Your choice of HT administration is personal. Do you prefer to take a pill once a day, put on a patch once or twice a week, apply daily gel or spray to your skin, or administer estrogen vaginally? We are all different. Talk to your practitioner and let her know what you prefer.

In large population studies, transdermal applications have been associated with lower risks of blood clots and strokes than standard doses of estrogen pills. When you take a pill it is processed through the liver. Transdermal options are absorbed by the skin, and so bypass the liver. Also, transdermal options can be prescribed in lower doses than pills, because they don't have to be digested.

If you are one of the 20% to 45% of midlife women suffering from vaginal symptoms (dryness or painful intercourse), vaginal application may be a good choice for you. The estrogen is delivered vaginally via creams or vaginal tablets (suppositories). You do not need to oppose the estrogen cream with progesterone, because the dose is so small that the only area treated is vaginal, and it is not absorbed significantly into your bloodstream. Vaginal HT application does not treat hot flashes and other menopause symptoms, just vaginal dryness.

Once you decide on your hormone recipe (ET or EPT), how you wish to take it (orally, transdermally or vaginally), and when you take it, your practitioner can prescribe the appropriate therapy, based on your needs and preferences.

TYPES OF HORMONES

In order to choose the right HT, it helps to understand the different types of hormones: how they are derived, how they are made and where. As I explain the different types of hormones, I'll clarify some of those confusing buzzwords for you—*natural, bioidenticals,* and *compounding.*

THE INGREDIENTS

In general, estrogen products are chemically synthesized, primarily from an active ingredient called diosgenin, a molecule extracted from the tubers and flowers of various plants including Dioscorea, a wild yam. Another source that is used to make conjugated estrogen, as I is found in Premarin, is isolated from the urine of pregnant mares. These sources are then synthesized--altered through biosynthetic manufacturing processes--to create a formulation that can be used to produce the actual pills, patches, creams, gels, or vaginal tablets.

Many of us want to use a "natural" product, since going through menopause is a natural transition. But you may be asking yourself, "How can the end product be 'natural' after it has been synthesized?" Sadly, the word *natural* is a marketing term. Some companies market their hormones as "natural" because the hormone used had a plant origin. However, all hormones, whether made in compounding pharmacies or in manufacturers' laboratories, are synthetic in the sense that they are made by chemical processes.

After the 2002 Women's Health Initiative (WHI) results (increase in breast cancer, heart attacks and strokes), many of us were afraid to use hormone therapy thinking it was harmful. That is when the word *natural* started being used to advertise hormones. *Natural* does not necessarily mean healthier and is primarily used for its advertising appeal.

HOW IT IS MADE

BIOIDENTICAL: A hormone manufactured in a laboratory that is chemically identical to the hormones produced by a woman's body. Bioidenticals are made of chemically altered ingredients from plant sources. Some believe a bioidentical hormone is a more "natural" option because it is the same molecular structure as our hormones, but the actual ingredients used in bioidenticals are synthesized (altered through chemical manufacturing processes) in a laboratory.

NONBIOIDENTICAL: A hormone manufactured in a laboratory that is not exactly chemically identical to the hormones produced by a woman's body. Nonbioidenticals also use synthesized ingredients derived from plant or animal sources.

WHERE ARE THEY MADE?

LABORATORY: A manufacturer's laboratory must abide by the FDA's rules and regulations. A hormone formulation created in a lab must follow FDA quality control on dosing and effectiveness. The ingredients and the process are FDA-approved. That means a lot of testing was done to make sure the treatment is safe for you. Your doctor can prescribe bioidentical HT produced in a regulated laboratory. Hormone products produced in a laboratory are also referred to as "conventional" therapy. Both bioidentical and non-bioidentical hormone therapies are produced in a regulated manufacturer's laboratory.

COMPOUNDING PHARMACY: Compounding pharmacies combine, mix, or alter ingredients to create a customized hormone for an individual patient. Unlike hormones that are made in a laboratory, compounding pharmacies have not demonstrated the safety, effectiveness and quality control with large, scientific studies that the FDA requires of standard pharmaceutical manufacturers. Compounding pharmacies use chemically synthesized hormones made from plants-- the same government-approved ingredients that are used in a manufacturer's laboratory. However, compounded "individualized" formulations are not necessarily uniform for purity, potency or efficiency. There is no registry of adverse effects from compounded medicines and there is no formal way to monitor adverse reactions.

A compounded formulation may benefit an individual who does not respond to conventional HT, or needs greater dosing flexibility needs to avoid allergens or needs treatment options where there is no commercial product available (such as testosterone). Compounding pharmacies are regulated by state pharmacy boards using U.S. Pharmacopeia (USP) standards - the official public standard setting authority for all prescriptions and over-the-counter medicines and dietary supplements – not federal FDA regulations.

Many women find compounded hormones appealing because they are marketed as a more "natural" option, but the ingredients are still the same synthesized hormones. I tried a common custom-compounded estrogen, and my estrogen levels went through the roof. When I had a hormone blood test, my estrogen levels were almost seven times higher than normal levels! I suspect the mixtures were inconsistent, and I was probably not giving myself the exact doses everyday. Using compounded hormones, made by your pharmacist and applied by you, leaves room for error. Mixing and application mistakes can dramatically affect you and your treatment results.

COMPOUNDING PHARMACY VERSUS LABORATORY

To better understand the differences, let's compare hormones that are made in a compounding pharmacy to conventional hormone therapy:

Compounding Pharmacy (bioidentical)	Conventional Laboratory (bioidentical and nonbioidentical)
Chemically identical to human hormones	Chemically identical or similar to human
Lack of FDA oversight	Has FDA oversight
Unmonitored doses; may be inaccurate and may be inconsistent	Monitored doses; accurate and consistent
Not FDA-tested; unknown risks	FDA-tested; known risks
Effectiveness unproven	Effectiveness tested and proven
Insufficient scientific evidence	Scientific evidence exists, and is conclusive evidence

Source: The Endocrine Society

HORMONE THERAPY FACTS

Ladies, these are the facts:

1. Compounding pharmacies and manufacturer's laboratories use the same ingredients.

2. There is no scientific evidence that custom-compounded bioidenticals are safer or more effective than standard pharmaceutical bioidentical prescriptions. There are no large, placebo-controlled studies to support claims of safety or effectiveness.

3. There are standard prescription formulations of bioidentical estradiol and micronized progesterone that are FDA-tested and approved. This type of prescription hormone therapy has been carefully standardized when it is manufactured. There are many standard FDA-approved bioidenticals available.

4. According to a recent online survey of U.S. pharmacists at compounding pharmacies, there are an estimated 26 to 33 million prescriptions a year for unregulated, non-FDA approved, compounded hormone therapy for women at menopause.

5. Both the compounding pharmacies and pharmaceutical industries promote their products. Bioidentical hormone therapy has provided the largest revenue stream of any compounded therapeutic drug category for the peri- and postmenopausal demographic.

6. Compounded bioidentical hormone therapy products do not have a "package insert" specifying risks or effectiveness, and they are not approved by the FDA.

7. An FDA survey (Center for Drug Evaluation and Research) ordered 29 products (various therapeutic uses and hormone therapies) from 12 compounding pharmacies and tested them. Thirty-four percent of these products failed at least one standard quality control test. Twenty-five percent failed potency standards among compounded hormones. When the FDA tested 3,000 pharmaceutical products there was only a failure rate of less than 2 percent for all tests.

So what does this all mean for you? Both compounding pharmacies and manufacturers' laboratories are essentially using the same ingredients. When choosing the hormone therapy that's right for you, keep in mind that both compounding and pharmaceutical companies are in the business of making money-- the word *natural* is a marketing term. Pharmaceutical companies must abide by strict FDA regulations to make sure your hormone products are safe and uniform, and the products were tested so you know your risks. Compounding pharmacies do not have the same restrictions.

DECIDING WHICH HORMONE THERAPY IS RIGHT FOR YOU

Your clinician will assess your individualized situation and prescribe the hormone therapy she thinks will best address your symptoms or health concerns. Understanding your hormone options helps you participate in that choice and find the approach that's best for you.

No single hormone recipe will work for every woman. You must take the time to work with your health-care practitioner to make adjustments. During one of our many conversations discussing hormone therapy, Dr. Klein said, "You cannot give every woman the same dress – she has to try it on to see if it fits. Sometimes you have to alter the dress, so it fits better." This same philosophy applies to hormone therapy, as it does to many medications. You start out with the lowest dose, and make adjustments if necessary. The exception to this rule is the woman who is in abrupt surgical menopause, in which case, it is generally necessary to start with the higher dose of HT, and taper down as tolerated.

MENOPAUSE MAKEOVER HORMONE THERAPY CHEAT SHEET

1. The only "natural" hormones are the hormones being made by your body.
2. Laboratories create molecules that are either identical (bioidentical) or not (non-bioidentical) to those in your body.
3. You have the choice to use a product that is regulated and tested or not.
4. Choose the product that works best for you. This may mean trying different doses or schedules or types until you find the right one.
5. Being informed is your first step to managing your menopause transition.

Review your symptoms and discuss your lifestyle with your doctor, so that you make the correct choices. If you decide hormone therapy is the best option for you, understand what you are taking, the side effects and the risks.

COMMON SIDE EFFECTS OF HT

HT can help you feel more like yourself again, but there are potential side effects that you should be aware of.

UTERINE BLEEDING, OR SPOTTING: If you experience this, you can try a lower estrogen dose. Most bleeding from hormone therapy subsides over time. Unexpected, unusually heavy or recurring bleeding needs to be evaluated by your health-care provider.

BREAST TENDERNESS: Try a lower estrogen dose; switch to another estrogen; limit salt intake; switch to another progestin; limit caffeine and chocolate. Generally, after three months it subsides once you are on an established hormone regimen.

NAUSEA: Nausea is uncommon but usually subsides once on an established regimen.

BLOATING: Try switching to low-dose, non-oral estrogen, lowering the progesterone dose to a level that still protects the uterus.

FLUID RETENTION: Limit salt intake.

HEADACHE/MIGRAINE: Switch to non-oral estrogen; lower the dose of estrogen and/or progesterone; switch to a continuous-combined regimen; switch to progesterone or a 19-norpregnane derivative; drink water, limit intake of salt, caffeine and alcohol.

MOOD CHANGES WITH EPT: Make sure you are not suffering from depression or anxiety; lower the progesterone dose; switch progesterone; change to a continuous-combined EPT regimen.

CORNEA SHAPE CHANGES: Unfortunately, no current solution strategy exists.

Good news—weight gain is *not* a side effect of hormone therapy!

IS HORMONE THERAPY SAFE?

There is a lot of confusion regarding the safety of HT. We have all seen the headlines and watched the news reports stating hormone therapy has risks. Before the 2002 Women's Health Initiative (WHI) report, many doctors treated menopausal women with HT, thinking the use of estrogen and progestin *after* menopause helped protect women against heart disease. But in 2002, the WHI came out with a study that found an increased risk of heart attack, stroke and breast cancer for women postmenopause. Headlines warned women against taking hormone therapy without fully disclosing all the facts and issues pertaining to this study. The HT public fear factor was so great that 56 percent of HT users aged 50 and older tried to discontinue therapy after this study. What was not revealed in those headlines was the WHI was not a study of treatment for menopausal symptoms. It was a study focused on determining whether HT prevented chronic illnesses. The average age of the participants was 63, with two-thirds of them starting hormone therapy more than ten years after menopause. Women with severe symptoms were generally not included in the WHI. A few years later, the WHI narrowed its focus on a second trial looking at the health effects of hormone therapy in younger (under 60 years old) verses older women. They found that younger postmenopausal women actually experienced *lower* risk of adverse health effects from hormone therapy than their older counterparts.

There have been many other studies focusing on HT and heart disease that revealed menopausal women between the ages of 50 and 59 who took HT for less than 10 years did not have an increased risk of heart disease. Women who began HT long after menopause had an increased risk of adverse effects.

Hormone therapy is still the most effective treatment for menopausal symptoms. Discuss your concerns with your practitioner, who can help you decide whether to take hormone therapy, and if so, at what age, the dosage, and for how long.

HORMONE THERAPY AND CANCER

Will hormone therapy increase your chance of cancer? The good news is that if taken in proper doses, for a limited period of time (less than 5 years), HT has not been reported to increase your risk of breast and uterine cancers. HT does not typically affect cervical, ovarian or lung cancer risks, especially when used for less than five years. Also, results from the WHI found that women on HT had a lower risk of colon cancer.

Throughout the past decade, research has consistently shown that HT is only a risk if taken for longer than 5 years or in high doses. The risk appears to be greater with combined estrogen and progestin regimens than with estrogen alone. Be sure to talk to your doctor about whether HT is safe for you, as the degree of risk is based on personal history, family history, and multiple other factors and must be evaluated on an individual, case-by-case basis.

Estrogen therapy (ET) and estrogen with progesterone therapy (EPT) can be a powerful tool in managing menopause –it helps relieve many symptoms. Since hormone therapy is prescribed at lower doses than in the past, it has fewer side effects. It is essential for each woman to weigh the individual benefits and risks of treatment. I personally found relief with hormone therapy. It also took a healthy eating plan, exercising most days of the week, and incorporating yoga (a complementary remedy) into my life to feel normal again.

IF HORMONE THERAPY IS NOT AN OPTION

Hormone therapy isn't always an option. If you're at risk for breast cancer, heart disease, uterine cancer, stroke, or deep vein thrombosis, or if you have a history of blood clotting, your clinician may advise you to consider other treatment options. Not to worry, you still have choices for treating symptoms.

ALTERNATIVES TO HORMONE THERAPY

Medication options

- Gabapentin (used for neurological purposes, to prevent seizures, and for chronic pain syndrome) may be used to treat hot flashes, particularly for those occurring at night and disturbing sleep
- Antidepressants to treat irritability and hot flashes
- Clonidine (blood pressure medication) is sometimes used to treat hot flashes. Possible side effects are dry mouth and sleep disturbances.

Lifestyle options

- Cardiovascular exercise 5 to 6 days per week
- Strength training 2-3 days per week
- Follow Menopause Makeover Food Pyramid (see page 51)
- No smoking
- Limited alcohol consumption
- Monitor blood pressure and cholesterol levels
- Layered clothing

Alternative & Complimentary options

- Calcium & Vitamin D for bone health
- Black cohosh (Remifemin is a popular standardized brand) used to treat hot flashes and night sweats (more information on herbal remedies on pages 27)
- Astroglide to treat vaginal dryness
- Practice relaxation techniques to manage hot flashes, sleep problems, moodiness (more on page 30)

COMPLEMENTARY AND ALTERNATIVE REMEDIES

Most of us would love to treat our menopause symptoms "naturally," since menopause is a "natural" event in our life. This involves using practices such as yoga and acupuncture and products, such as herbs or phytoestrogens that are not used by conventional medical practitioners. Complementary and alternative medicine (CAM) incorporates a variety of healing philosophies, therapies and approaches not conventionally used by the Western medical community. A treatment or remedy is *complementary* when it is used with *conventional* (mainstream medical community) therapies. *Alternative* remedies are used instead of conventional treatment. According to the National Institutes of Health (NIH), over 36 percent of Americans use some form of CAM. If you decide to use CAM to treat your menopause symptoms, you're not alone.

PHYTOESTROGENS AND HERBAL TREATMENTS

Women have used herbs to treat menopause symptoms for years. If you are going to use herbal remedies, be sure to use products manufactured by reputable firms to avoid unregulated production standards or contamination. Alternative remedies do not have the U.S. Food and Drug Administration's (FDA) stamp of approval and are not usually covered by insurance. Scientific tests or trials on many alternative products, such as herbs, may not exist. Also be aware that long-term safety data is lacking in herbal use.

The National Center for Complementary and Alternative Medicine (NCCAM) at the NIH stimulates, develop and support research on CAM. In Canada the National Health Products Directorate

(NHPD) regulates CAM products. If your symptoms are mild and you choose CAM therapies to treat your symptoms, work closely with a health-care practitioner to ensure safe therapy. Many of these therapies can be controversial. It is important to discuss all "natural" remedies with your doctor, as some herbal products can be dangerous if they are taken with other drugs. CAM therapies may not treat severe menopause symptoms, and cannot treat osteoporosis and other diseases.

Phytoestrogens

INFORMATION: Phytoestrogens are plant-derived compounds with estrogen-like biologic activity and a chemical structure similar to estradiol. You can find phytoestrogens in isoflavones (soybeans and soy products) and lignans (flax seed). Soy is also a wonderful source of protein, omega-3 fatty acids, and it contains calcium. Soybeans, soy flour, miso soup, tempeh, tofu, tofu yogurt, soy hot dog, soymilk and soy sauce all contain isoflavone content. Apples, basil, barley, green tea, garlic, licorice, corn, parsley, and sesame seeds also contain phytoestrogens.

USES: Many women use phytoestrogens to relieve symptoms such as hot flashes, night sweats, vaginal dryness, and to improve cognitive function. Evidence regarding the effectiveness for hot flashes is mixed.

WARNINGS: Not every woman's body can convert soy isoflavones into the plant-derived form of estrogen. Soy's possible role in breast cancer is uncertain. If you are at risk of developing breast cancer or other hormone-sensitive conditions (ovarian or uterine cancer), discuss with your practitioner.

Black Cohosh

INFORMATION: One of the most popular herbal treatments for menopause is Black Cohosh, because many believe it has estrogen-like activity. But recent research suggests that black cohosh acts more like a SERM ("Selective Estrogen Receptor Modulator" compounds that bind with estrogen receptors exhibiting estrogen action in some tissues and anti-estrogen action in other tissues) than an estrogen. Recently, the FDA required cautionary statements due to some reports of liver toxicity from excessive black cohosh use.

USES: Many women take this herb to treat hot flashes, night sweats, vaginal dryness, stress, arthritis, and muscle pain. Studies of its effectiveness in reducing hot flashes have yielded mixed results despite claims women get hot flash relief from black cohosh.

SIDE EFFECTS: include gastrointestinal discomfort, headaches, nausea, vomiting and dizziness.

WARNINGS: Black cohosh has salicylate in it, so do not take it if you are taking aspirin or other blood thinners.

Chasteberry

INFORMATION: Also known as monk's pepper and sage tree hemp, chasteberry was used in the Middle Ages to decrease sexual desire.

USES: Women have reported improvements in mood, headaches and breast tenderness; but scientific evidence is lacking.

Side effects: include GI problems, acne-like rashes and dizziness.

Warnings: Chasteberry may affect certain hormone levels. Do not take chasteberry if you are taking birth-control pills. Chasteberry may also affect the dopamine system in the brain, so avoid if you are using amantadine, levodopa or SSRIs ("selective serotonin reuptake inhibitors," a class of antidepressants).

Valerian Root

Information: Valerian root was historically used to treat insomnia.

Uses: A sleep aid, and to treat nervousness, depression, headaches, irregular heartbeat, and anxiety. Valerian improves sleep when taken nightly for one to two weeks.

Side effects: include headaches, dizziness, upset stomach and tiredness the morning after use.

Warning: Valerian root can give you a hangover feeling, so use with caution.

Dong Quai

Information: Also known as tang gui.

Uses: A blood-thinner, and to treat hot flashes and cramps.

Warnings: Although taken to reduce hot flashes, but studies found it was no better than a placebo. Dong Quai contains compounds that can thin the blood, and it makes the skin more sensitive to the sun, so beware this herb can be potentially toxic. Women with fibroids, hemophilia or other blood-clotting problems should not use dong quai.

Ginseng

Information: American ginseng is similar to Asian ginseng, *Panax ginseng*, L., which grows wild in Northern Manchuria.

Uses: Relieves stress, mood symptoms, sleep disturbances, can stimulate a low sex drive and boost immunity. Ginseng has not been found to be helpful for treatment of hot flashes. Some claim it can lower blood glucose and control blood pressure.

Side effects: include nervousness, insomnia, headaches, GI problems, dizziness, hypertension, and can cause allergic reaction. Asian ginseng may lower levels of blood sugar. So if you have diabetes, use caution.

Warnings: Ginseng has been found to inhibit platelet aggregation (blood clotting). Warning - do not combine with an anticoagulant, aspirin or vitamin E.

Ginkgo Biloba

Information: A blood-thinner and antioxidant.

Uses: Has been used to improve memory and sense of well-being, although recent studies suggest that the use of ginkgo biloba does not improve memory.

Side effects: include headache, GI distress, diarrhea, dizziness, or allergic skin reactions.

Warnings: Do not combine with an anticoagulant, aspirin or vitamin E.

Red Clover

INFORMATION: Contains estrogen-like compounds.

USES: Relieves menopausal symptoms (hot flashes, vaginal dryness, mood swings), high cholesterol, and osteoporosis. Some women claim red clover can reduce hot flashes, but scientific evidence is lacking.

SIDE EFFECTS: Studies report few side effects and no serious health problems.

St. John's Wort

INFORMATION: Some say the name *St. John's Wort* refers to John the Baptist, as the plant blooms around the time of the feast of St. John the Baptist in late June.

USES: A popular treatment for anxiety, sleep disorders, mild to moderate depression, and nerve pain. Some women take St. John's Wort with black cohosh to relieve hot flashes, but scientific evidence is lacking.

SIDE EFFECTS: Dry mouth, GI upset, headache, dizziness, nausea, fatigue, and sexual dysfunction.

WARNINGS: St. John's Wort has significant drug interactions, so it is important to discuss this herb's use with your healthcare provider. Do not take St. John's Wort with SSRIs, birth control pills, or warfarin (blood thinners). Take with food to avoid stomach upset. St. John's Wort may cause increased sensitivity to sunlight.

ALTERNATIVE PRACTICES

Alternative practices are often used to help alleviate menopausal symptoms. Many women find that they help, although according to the National Center for Complementary and Alternative Medicine, continued research is needed to determine their effectiveness. At this time, there is not enough strong scientific evidence to recommend the use of botanicals, according to NCCAM, the think tank at the NIH.

ACUPUNCTURE: Traditional Chinese Medicine (TCM) corrects energy imbalances using needles properly placed in various parts of your body. Some women claim they get menopausal relief from acupressure and/or acupuncture. Because needles are used to perform acupuncture, hire a qualified specialist.

MASSAGE: Oriental massage is used to bring the body back into harmony. This is one of my favorite alternative practices.

YOGA: Yoga is a wonderful activity to add to your exercise and stress-management plan.

It helps to relieve stress, prevent osteoporosis, reduce mood swings, increase strength and flexibility, and improve self-esteem.

MEDITATION AND BREATHING EXERCISES: Believed to help calm the mind and body, resulting in self-acceptance and a sense of well-being.

AYURVEDA: India's traditional system of medicine, emphasizing equal balance between the mind, body and spirit to achieve harmony. Treatments include exercise, diet, meditation, massage, herbs, and controlled breathing.

MIND-BODY MEDICINE: Hypnosis, biofeedback, music, dance, prayer, visual imagery, meditation, and art therapy are forms of mind-body medicine. Biofeedback has had some success controlling hot flashes and stress incontinence.

REFLEXOLOGY: The foot and sometimes the hand are massaged with pressure applied to *reflex* zones to restore proper balance and remove unhealthy blockages.

ENERGY MEDICINE: Reiki, gi gong and healing touch are therapies that focus on energy fields within the body or from outside sources.

COMBINATION OF TREATMENT OPTIONS

Be prepared to try a number of options before you have success. If you are like me, you will need to be patient and continue to search for the correct treatment option until you find one that works for you. Discuss your symptoms and treatment options with your health-care provider. Perhaps a combination of hormone therapy and complementary practices may bring you relief, as it did for me.

Remember, being informed is an asset during your menopause transition—keep up-to-date on the latest research and keep track of your symptoms over time. As your symptoms change, you will most likely need to adjust your approach.

MAKEOVER TIPS

* Surround yourself with loved ones who support you.
* Become informed.
* Make lifestyle changes.
* Develop a partnership with your doctor or practitioner.
* Document your symptoms.
* If you choose to use hormone therapy, it should be based on your individual needs and medical history.

MAKEOVER TAKE ACTION LIST

* Document your symptoms (intensity and date) in your Symptom Checklist in Chapter 1.
* Visit your healthcare provider and request a FSH blood test. Prepare ahead of time with the "Make the Most of Your Doctor's Visit" tips on page 7.
* What type of treatment course have you chosen to discuss with your doctor?
* Record your course of action to managing menopause symptoms under *hormones* in Chapter 12.

IN YOUR ESSENTIAL PLANNER

* Record your appointments (doctor, practitioner, lab tests, medical tests) in Your Month-at-a-Glance Planner.
* Record your hormone treatment and dosage each day (alternative or medical) in Your 12-Week Plan.
* Record any other medications you may be taking (blood pressure medication, cholesterol medication, antibiotics, aspirin, allergy medication) in Your 12-Week Plan.
* Document your symptoms daily in Your 12-Week Plan (hot flashes, night sweats, irregular periods, loss of libido). Are there patterns with your symptoms?
* Record your emotional and physical concerns in your Journal
* How you feel each day is important. Note your feelings each day in Your 12-Week Plan.
* Record your weekly progress, noting symptoms in Your12-Week Plan.
* Keep track of your support team in Your Menopause Makeover Contacts
* Complete the Menopause Makeover Medical Forms

| Chapter 3 | Step Two: Feeding the New You How Food Can Set You Free! |

Having always been one of the lucky ones who could eat anything without gaining a pound, I felt as if menopause tackled me from behind and tossed me into the air like a rag doll. I plummeted to earth, weighing an extra 25 pounds and measuring an additional 17 inches, in less than six months!

I ran to the nearest bookstore and purchased diet books, ordered expensive pre-made diet food, called friends who were diet experts, and subscribed to online diet programs – all to no avail. After months of failure, the only thing I had lost was control of my life.

Hopeless, I surrendered to my never-ending menopausal food cravings. Every afternoon, I sat in front of the television watching *Oprah*, eating a slab of Brie cheese, and nursing a bottle of red wine to numb my dismay at being so overweight. My poor fiancé witnessed his fun, sexy, independent bride-to-be fall into a hellish abyss of self-pity. Even his unconditional love and support could not save me when I was in this condition.

I have always been able to rescue myself, but menopause pushed every dysfunctional button I had. I lost control over my body, my self-confidence, and my life. I struggled with the fact that I was aging, and I could not stop it. I felt a sense of failure in my relationship with my future husband. I worried that I could no longer bear children, even though we didn't plan on having any. It became clear to me, or so I thought, that "the change" really meant "the end."

Those feelings added a hefty 25 pounds to my small frame in less than six months. I was living in a self-imposed "fat suit," hiding under baggy clothes, hoping no one would notice. My former self was screaming to get out.

Terrified that I would walk down the aisle looking like an over-stuffed sausage, I made a startling discovery. My weight loss goals were focused on the perception that I was not perfect. I thought I had to lose weight in order to find my perfect self again, as opposed to acknowledging that I was already perfect, just buried under a "fat suit." This fat suit was built on the fear of aging, hormonal cravings, midlife stress, and far too many cookies, ice cream, cheese and wine. I was feeding an unhealthy body thousands of extra calories a day, fueling extra weight gain and unhappiness. Once I revised my goals so that I was feeding and nurturing the already perfect me that existed under my menopause fat suit, the perfect me re-emerged! I did not have to search for my healthy weight. It already existed!

I started taking care of the perfect me, feeding her the food she needed to be healthy – and exercising. Those extra 2,000 calories I was consuming daily while watching *Oprah* had produced a very impressive fat suit. (Note to Oprah: Your show gave me comfort; unfortunately so did the Brie cheese!)

Once I calculated the calories I needed to feed my healthy size, and redefined the food ratios I needed to consume, the zipper on the fat suit started unzipping. As motivation, I printed out copies of an "inspirational picture" of myself at my healthy weight – taken just two years earlier – that I placed on my desk and exercise machine. Three months later, and 25 pounds lighter, the healthy me emerged.

Eating the correct foods in the proper portions actually helped alleviate many of my miserable menopause symptoms. Food had set me free!

In this chapter, I will review important information regarding food so that you understand how to eat right for your changing body. Armed with the facts, you can set your weight-loss and nutrition goals in Part Two of the book and create a personal food plan to achieve those goals in Part Three.

A majority of women ages 45-55 will gain weight. . During menopause, it is natural for the body to store some fat around your "middle," so that your waistline starts to disappear. It is normal to gain five to ten pounds during menopause, but it's really your *lifestyle* habits that cause you to gain weight. That's good news—it means that with small adjustments to your diet and exercise habits, you can outsmart menopause and keep your waistline trim!

Weight gain is often one of the most frustrating symptoms we experience during menopause. You may notice the fat around your hips, thighs and rear shifting upwards to your mid-section. You may feel discouraged because weight loss methods that worked before menopause no longer work. The good news is that five to ten pounds of weight gain during "the change" reflects a readjustment of your metabolism, and you can learn to live with this. However, beyond that, you are probably not being rigorous about watching your caloric intake or exercising sufficiently to balance your intake.

Going through so many changes during menopause will force you to look at your health, emotions, and lifestyle choices. If you have gained an excessive amount of weight, understanding how your body is changing will give you the tools to manage your weight during menopause. Menopausal weight gain is a wake-up call to eat delicious, healthy food, and enjoy a more active lifestyle.

FEED THE HEALTHY YOU.

WHY YOU GAIN WEIGHT DURING MENOPAUSE

A number of factors can contribute to that extra belly bulge during menopause.

THE PHYSICAL

TESTOSTERONE: Testosterone is a hormone produced by the ovaries and adrenal glands that is 50 to 60 percent lower by the time your go through menopause. When levels of testosterone decrease, your metabolism slows.

GENETICS: Look at your family tree. Are there members who carry excessive weight around the abdomen? Genetics may also be a factor affecting weight gain.

SLOWER METABOLISM: Your metabolism slows as you age, so you cannot eat the same size portions as you were younger. If you do, you will likely gain weight.

MEDICAL CONDITIONS: Medical conditions such as insulin resistance (when your body becomes resistant to the insulin it produces) or an underactive thyroid can cause weight gain or even certain medications can cause you to gain weight. Speak to your doctor if you think this is a possibility.

LIFESTYLE CHOICES

UNHEALTHY EATING: Many women with busy schedules do not have the time to prepare healthy meals with appropriate portions. Eating fast food, and comfort foods in large portions, will only contribute to weight gain.

NOT EXERCISING OR EXERCISING LESS: Most women taking care of a family, partner, and parents are also balancing a career at the same time. It is understandable that making time to exercise takes a back seat to other priorities. During perimenopause through postmenopause, incorporating exercise into your daily routine is critical to being healthy. (More on exercise in Chapter 4.)

10 WAYS TO COPE WITH STRESS

1. Identify stress factors in your home life, work situation, schedule, and lifestyle.

2. Relax. Spend 20 quiet minutes a day. Pray, meditate, do relaxation visualization exercises.

3. Communicate with loved ones. Ask for support.

4. Create a plan to resolve your stressful situations.

5. Incorporate exercise into your routine. Get physical. Start a garden. Take daily walks.

6. Watch your food intake. Try to eat healthy foods and eliminate fast foods. Avoid excessive caffeine, alcohol, sugar, and absolutely avoid tobacco.

7. Focus attention on time management. Do essential tasks and prioritize other activities. Don't try to do everything at once.

8. Get enough sleep. Pamper yourself.

9. Take a vacation. Go somewhere you have always dreamed of going.

10. Decide to be happy, love yourself, laugh, and remember no one is perfect.

MEDICATIONS

PRESCRIPTION DRUGS: Some prescription drugs, such as antidepressants, can contribute to weight gain.

If you started gaining weight after beginning a new prescription, discuss with your health-care provider. Do not stop taking your medications without a conversation with your doctor or clinician.

THE EMOTIONAL

Emotional eating is very common—many people eat when they feel sad, lonely, or stressed. But you don't have to let emotional eating sabotage your Menopause Makeover! The first step to conquering emotional eating is awareness.

ARE YOU AN EMOTIONAL EATER?

Did your parents give you food as a reward when you were a child?
Are you frustrated with something in your life?
Are you bored with your life or someone in your life?
Are you sad about a situation in your life?
Are you lonely?

If you answered, "yes" to at least three of these questions, you may be an emotional eater. As women, we are emotional creatures. Many of us eat to find comfort. Living in a society where women have careers, families, homes and financial responsibilities – no wonder we are grabbing brownies and cupcakes!

STRESS: THE DIET SABOTEUR

When your body is under stress, the hormone cortisol tells your body to go into *storage mode* for survival. Your body thinks it is in trouble and starts storing calories, causing weight gain. Stress hormones may block weight loss. You can experience stress from daily emotional events, dieting, lack of sleep from night sweats, and depression. If you have unresolved emotional issues, they may surface during your menopause transition. This type of cortisol-induced stress can lead to food cravings, overeating, a slower metabolism, fluctuating blood sugar levels, and fat storage around the waistline. If you are struggling with weight issues, take a look at the levels of stress in your life.

HIDING UNDER A FAT SUIT

As we get older, we start noticing the effects of aging, we experience weight gain, and many of us struggle with the reality that having children is no longer possible. For many, these changes can affect our self-esteem. When we don't feel good about ourselves, it is common for us to overeat, and stop taking care of our health in general – both physical and emotional. Often we start to feel "safe" hiding under a self-imposed fat suit.

One of the first-steps to living your perfect weight is addressing unresolved emotional issues. When you commit intellectually and emotionally to living your perfect weight, the rest of the journey is the execution of your menopause weight management plan.

Why are you hiding under a fat suit?

10 WAYS TO CONQUER EMOTIONAL EATING

1. Identify what feelings come up for you when you reach for a pint of ice cream.

2. If bored, find an activity you can do when you feel emotional and start craving sugar, alcohol or salty foods. Take a walk, clean the house, work in your garden, or call a friend.

3. When you feel emotional eating taking over during a stressful situation, close your eyes, breathe deeply and think of someone who loves you or whom you love. Every inhalation breathe in *love*, every exhalation breathe out *stress*. Fill yourself with *love*, not ice cream.

4. If lonely, find a buddy who also struggles with emotional eating and create a support team.

5. Start a daily journal and record your feelings when you feel the urge to eat.

6. If you're overworked and feeling exhausted, remember to make time for yourself: Take a nap, make time to exercise or take a yoga class.

7. If you're anxious, think about why this might be. Are you are drinking too much coffee? Stressed at work? Identify the trigger and work to lessen the stress.

8. If feeling frustrated with a life situation or person, confront it or them and find a way to deal with it. Can you find a solution for the situation challenging you? If someone is driving you crazy, try to stand in the other person's shoes and be positive, and create healthy boundaries. Instead of complaining about a situation or person, search for a life lesson to learn and then move on.

9. Remove tempting food from your house and office. This way you're more apt to eat when you are hungry not emotional.

10. If emotional eating, stress, depression, or anxiety becomes a larger issue, seek professional help.

There are many logical explanations for gaining weight during menopause. Whether physical, emotional or lifestyle choices, understanding the causes allow you to conquer and manage unwanted and unhealthy weight.

FOOD CAN SET YOU FREE

After you address any unresolved emotional issues that may be contributing to your weight gain, the next important factor in managing weight is learning how food can set you free. There are three categories of food: proteins, fats and carbohydrates. In order to maintain health, you need to consume nutrients from all three of these categories.

PROTEIN IS THE HERO

The word *protein* is derived from a Greek root meaning "of first importance." Your muscles, organs, bones, cartilage, antibodies, skin, some hormones, and all enzymes are made of protein.

Consuming the correct amount of protein has important benefits

1. Protein (chicken, turkey, beef, fish and beans) is digested more slowly from the stomach to the intestine. This makes you feel full longer. Protein does not stimulate the release of insulin so it helps stabilize blood sugar.
2. Consuming protein low in saturated fat can improve your blood triglycerides and high-density lipoprotein. This can reduce your risk of heart attack or stroke.
3. Protein is indispensable for the growth and maintenance of the cells in our body.
4. Our body development, healing of wounds, replacement of dead cells, hair and nail growth and the replenishment of lost blood is dependant on protein.
5. Proteins in the form of enzymes, antibodies and hormones can promote a strong healthy metabolic process, and boost your nervous and immunity systems.

Not consuming enough protein can lead to weakening of the muscles, heart and respiratory system: impaired growth, decreased immunity, and even death. As you go through menopause, protein is the hero –it keeps your body from clinging to fat.

SOY IS A STAR

Soy is a wonderful source of protein. The *Archives of Internal Medicine* found a link between soy consumption and strong bones. Women who consumed 13 grams per day of soy had 35 to 37 percent lower risk of fractures compared to women in the lowest intake group. Soy also contains other wonderful nutrients, such as omega-3 fatty acids, fiber and B vitamins. If you do not consume meats or other animal products, soy protein is a healthy alternative. Both the American Dietetic Association and the Food and Drug Administration confirm that people who eat 25 to 50 grams of soy protein per day can help lower their levels of LDL cholesterol ("bad" cholesterol that can clog blood vessels).

Other yummy non-meat sources of protein are beans and legumes, nuts, peanut butter, cheese, whole grain products and yogurt.

COMPLETE VS. INCOMPLETE PROTEINS

Not all proteins are created equally. Proteins consumed from animal sources (meat, fish, poultry, milk, cheese and eggs) are *complete proteins*. They contain all essential nine amino acids for human use. The only exception is soy (a plant source); it is also considered a complete protein. Amino acids are the chemical building blocks from which new proteins are made. Consuming complete proteins is important. Proteins obtained from plant-based foods (grains/cereals, legumes, seeds, nuts, lentils, peas and beans) are *incomplete proteins*. They do not possess the necessary amounts of essential amino acids for human use.

Why does this matter? If you are fulfilling a protein serving by consuming only nuts, it is not a *complete* protein. You need to have a variety of incomplete proteins to make up a complete protein. You can combine plant and animal foods, or plant proteins from a variety of grains and cereals for one meal or eat them separately at another meal to honor a complete daily protein serving.

HOW PROTEIN CAN BURN THAT BELLY FAT

For your Menopause Makeover, it's important to eat plenty of protein—a source of protein at every meal and snack. You should consume protein five to six times per day. The portion should be the size of the palm of your hand, around four to six ounces.

PERFECT PROTEINS FOR YOUR MENOPAUSE MAKEOVER

Choose Lean, Low-fat Protein Sources

Fish & Seafood	Salmon Cod Crab	Trout Tuna (canned in water) Shrimp
Poultry	*Remove the skin before cooking.* Chicken, light meat	 Turkey breast
Milk, Cheese and Yogurt *Dairy foods are excellent sources of protein, and they also contain calcium.*	*Skim or low fat dairy can help keep bones strong:* Cottage cheese Skim milk *Low-fat cheeses:* Swiss Jarlsberg Farmer's cheeses Romano Parmesan	 Yogurt Mozzarella Ricotta Provolone Feta Goat cheeses

Eggs	*You can eat egg whites daily – much lower in calories and fat than if you include the yolks.* Egg (medium) Egg whites
Legumes and Nuts	*Legumes and nuts are loaded with fiber, helping you feel full for hours.* Lima beans Almonds Lentils Cashews Peanut butter
Soy	*Soy protein can help lower cholesterol and reduce the risk of heart disease.* Soybeans Tofu
Lean Beef	Ground beef Sirloin steak
Protein Snacks On-the-go	Great protein snacks include: cereal bar, energy bar, or meal replacement drinks.

Menopause Makeover Planner Entry:
Go to the shopping list in the ultimate planner in Chapter
13 and check off your favorite *healthy* protein choices.

FAT: THE GOOD, THE BAD AND THE UGLY

Fat, like protein, is vital to your health. In moderate amounts fat transports oxygen to every cell in your body. Fat is a component for building cells, body tissue and absorbing some vitamins and other nutrients. It is also an essential component maintaining hormones, brain and nervous system.

CONSUMING THE CORRECT AMOUNT OF FAT HAS BENEFITS

* Fat provides energy for your body to stay warm. Excess calories are stored in fat deposits that insulate the body.

* Fat helps protect your body from injury.

* Fat helps maintain healthy skin.

* Fats can help the body process proteins and carbohydrates.

* Eating food with fat can help us feel a sense of fullness.

* The texture of fat can make food taste creamy and smooth and carry flavor.

* Fats regulate cholesterol metabolism.

* Fat carries fat-soluble vitamins such as vitamins A, D, E, and K by assisting in the absorption from the intestines.

* Fat cushions our vital organs, like the kidneys.

* Consuming fat is important for normal brain development.

* Fat is a secondary source of energy.

Consuming the correct type of fat, in the proper quantities, has some excellent benefits. There are three naturally occurring types of fats (monounsaturated, polyunsaturated, and saturated), and one human-made fat: (trans fat).

THE GOOD FATS
The good news is we can include good fats in our diet.

Monounsaturated Fats
The healthiest fat choice is monounsaturated fats. Olive oil, canola oil, peanut oil, macadamia oil, almonds, peanuts, pecans, cashews, and avocados contain monounsaturated fats. Vegetable oil fats remain liquid at room temperature, and are one of the healthiest oils to add to your food plan. Monounsaturated fats can lower your bad cholesterol (LDL) levels, and increase your good cholesterol (HDL) levels. I want to repeat this because it is so important: Monounsaturated fats help increase good cholesterol and lower bad cholesterol! Stock your house with olive oil, almonds and avocados.

Polyunsaturated Fats
Polyunsaturated fat is found in fish (salmon, halibut, herring and mackerel), soybeans, fish oils, and grain products. It is essential in our diet because polyunsaturated fat includes essential fatty acids— omega-3 and omega-6 — that our body cannot make for itself. Polyunsaturated fats can help lower the level of bad cholesterol (LDL).

Omega-3 fats can be found in fish oil. Polyunsaturated fish oils can protect the heart by lowering triglyceride levels and preventing blood clots. Natural sources of omega-3 are salmon, sardines, herring, and rainbow trout.

If you are not a fish lover, you can also find omega-3 in flaxseed, canola and soy oils, plus flax seeds, soybeans, pumpkin seeds, and walnuts.

Omega-6 can be found in soybean oil, corn oil, sunflower oil and cottonseed oil, and there are unproven claims that it is good for your skin and hair, and even with emotional health. However, omega-6 should be taken in moderation, because consuming high levels of omega-6 can interfere with the known omega-3's health benefits. Recent studies suggest that higher levels of omega-6 may increase the risk of other diseases and can contribute to depression. Omega-6 found in vegetable oils may even contribute to an increased breast cancer risk in postmenopausal women.

A typical "western diet" consumes a ratio of ten to one (10:1) of omega-6 to omega-3, often as high as 30:1. This high level of omega-6 limits the health benefits of omega-3. According to The National Institutes of Health and the U.S. National Library of Medicine state, both omega-3 and omega-6 must work in balance to benefit your health. Aim for a 4:1 ratio or lower for optimum benefits.

THE BAD FATS

Just as there are good fats, there are bad fats. Bad fats include: refined oils, partially hydrogenated oils, shortening, and commercially deep-fried foods. Fat is a concentrated source of calories, so we must closely monitor our intake. A diet too high in fat is linked to higher risk of weight gain, high blood pressure, certain cancers, and insulin resistance, as well as gallbladder disease.

Saturated fat

Saturated fat is found in red meat and other animal products such as dairy products (includ-ing cheese, sour cream, ice cream, butter), lard, and tropical oils such as coconut oil and coconut milk, cocoa butter, and palm oils. Saturated fats remain solid at room temperature. Saturated fats raise LDL (bad) cholesterol, which can lead to hardening of the arteries, and they contribute to blood clots. Blood clots can lead to clogged blood vessels that can result in a stroke or heart attack. When you purchase cheese, ice cream, sour cream and other dairy products, be sure to select low-fat options.

Trans Fat

Trans fat is a human-made fat, created by adding hydrogen to a polyunsaturated fat, turning liquid oils into more solid fats like margarine. Trans fats can be found in baked goods, fried foods, donuts, French fries, crackers and snacks. Trans fats raise your LDL (bad) cholesterol levels, and lower HDL (good) cholesterol levels, and increase your risk of heart disease. THis is a double-whammy bad fat choice! THe American Heart Association recommends an intake of no more than one percent of total trans fat calories per day.

THE UGLY

Since fat takes longer to digest than either protein or carbohydrates, you feel full longer after eating it. Yes, that fried chicken and bag of French fries will fill you up!

Many health organizations recommend consuming no more than 30 percent fat per day. During menopause your body is clinging to fat. For your *Menopause Makeover*, I suggest a daily calorie intake of 25 percent fat, with the emphasis on *good* fats.

MAKEOVER TIPS:

- Replace butter with olive oil.
- If you eat red meat, consume leaner cuts: pork loin, pork tenderloin, fresh ham, extra-lean ground beef.
- Consume lean meats: chicken without the skin, turkey, fish.
- Broil, bake, or grill to cook meat. If you need to fry, use a non-stick pan with only a small amount of vegetable oil spray.

CHART OF GOOD FAT SOURCES

Flax seed	Flaxseed oil	Safflower oil
Cashews	Sunflower oil	Soybean oil
Sunflower seeds	Pumpkin oil	Macadamia oils
Olive oil	Canola oil	Salmon
Peanut oil	Rainbow trout	Crab, blue
Halibut	Flounder	Herring
Haddock	Mackerel	Avocado
Sardines	Tuna	Peanuts
Olives	Soybeans	Pecans
Almonds	Walnuts	

Menopause Makeover Planner Entry:
Select healthy fat sources from this chart and enter
them in your "shopping list" in Chapter 13.

THE TRUTH ABOUT CARBOHYDRATES

Carbohydrates are an important part of a healthy diet. Without any carbohydrates in your diet you could feel fatigued, have muscle cramps, and suffer from poor mental function. Who needs poor mental function when you are going through menopause?

Carbohydrates, also known as "carbs," provide the body with fuel for physical activities and for proper organ function. Your body breaks down carbs, and turns them into glucose. We often refer to glucose as blood sugar. As we get older, and experience the menopause transition, not all carbs are "friendly" to our food plan. Most carbohydrates provide comfort, so many of us grab comfort carbs when suffering with menopause symptoms. It is critical to make healthy carb choices during your menopause transition. Understanding the difference between "good" and "bad" carbs can be an important step to gaining control over your menopause symptoms, such as weight gain, and overall health.

Consuming the *good* carbohydrates can:

* Provide easily obtained energy for your cells, tissues and organs.

* Provide essential vitamins and minerals.

* Provide an excellent source of fiber.

* Aid digestion and help your body reserve energy.

* Benefit muscle tissue.

* Benefit blood sugar levels because good carbs break down slowly, so glucose is released gradually into your system.

* Improve mental concentration.

* Improve your mood.

Complex Carbohydrates

Complex carbs are commonly known as "starches" like whole grain breads, cereals, brown rice, pasta, potatoes, bagels, starchy vegetables (corn, peas), and legumes (beans, lentils). Complex carbs take the body longer to digest because they are made up of chains of glucose molecules. The digestive system has to work harder to break down this chain into individual sugars so your body can absorb. Since complex carbs take longer to digest, they give you energy that lasts longer. Complex carbs often provide fiber. Wonderful carbs that can also provide fiber are fruits, vegetables and whole grains, whole grain bread, and whole grain pastas and cereals. These are "friendly" carbs, if consumed in moderation.

Simple Carbohydrates

Simple carbohydrates have smaller molecules of sugar, unlike the long chains of glucose found in complex carbs, and are digested quickly. Many products processed and prepared with refined sugar are simple carbs (white sugar, pastas, white bread, cakes, chocolate, biscuits). These are not "friendly" carbs for gals struggling with menopausal weight gain and fluctuating hormones, because they absorb quickly increasing the chances of the sugar being converted to fat. But fruits that are *natural* simple carbohydrates are high in fiber, like apples, pears, oranges, and strawberries, can actually help slow digestion decreasing the surge of sugar energy into your cells when its not needed, so the chance of it converting to fat decreases.

Other simple carbs are dairy products. Low-fat dairy products are healthy choices for your Menopause Makeover.

BLOOD SUGAR – THE UPS AND DOWNS

The Glycemic Index

Once we consume carbs, our body converts these carbs to energy very differently depending on whether they are simple or complex carbs. Understanding this difference can help you conquer unwanted weight gain.

The Glycemic Index (GI) is a scale that ranks carbohydrate-rich foods by based on how quickly and how high they boost blood sugar compared to pure glucose. The glycemic index number is the average amount that a particular food raises blood sugar levels. Eating high-glycemic foods (simple carbs) like white bread, soda, pasta dishes, chocolate bars, and potatoes can cause dramatic peaks in your blood sugar. Eating low-glycemic foods (complex carbs) like breakfast cereals (made of wheat bran, oats and/or barley), lentils, soybeans, baked beans, and fruit causes a more gentle change in blood sugar. Eating low-glycemic foods can help you manager your weight, prevent insulin resistance, and control type 2 diabetes.

Benefits of low-glycemic carbohydrates

- Stabilize blood sugar levels in your body that are sustained for longer periods of time.
- Your hunger urges are controlled because the blood sugar levels are more slowly. being released into your bloodstream.
- You are able to exercise for longer periods of time.
- Your risk of getting type 2 diabetes is lowered.
- Your risk of getting heart disease is lowered.
- Most low-glycemic foods are lower in calories and fat.
- Many low-glycemic foods are loaded with fiber and nutrients.
- Can help you lose weight during menopause.

All carbohydrates are broken down into simple sugars during digestion. This activates the production of insulin in your pancreas. As blood sugar levels increase, cells in the pancreas create more insulin to absorb the blood sugar. When this happens, the sugar levels in your bloodstream start falling. Then your pancreas starts making a hormone called glucagons to signal the liver to start releasing stored sugar. When this process is working properly, your body and brain have healthy levels of blood sugar.

When the cells do not respond to the insulin signal to receive sugar, insulin resistance can occur. Insulin resistance causes your blood sugar and insulin levels to stay high long after eating, thus causing the production of insulin to slow down or even stop

Insulin resistance can be dangerous to your health. It can increase your risk of type 2 diabetes, some cancers and heart disease.

Fortunately cutting down on the consumption of refined grains, and/or replacing them in your diet with whole grains, and consuming low-glycemic carbs can decrease your chance of insulin resistance and help you achieve a healthy weight.

THE GI AND YOUR HORMONES

Your food choices can make a drastic difference in your menopause symptoms. Eating a high-glycemic diet can affect the way your hormones are metabolized by slowing the production of estrogen from the adrenal glands. This is the last thing you want when your estrogen is naturally declining! Ever-changing hormones and stressful midlife changes can affect the way your body regulates insulin. Eating low to medium glycemic foods can help regulate insulin. Maintaining balanced blood sugar levels can help limit over stimulation of the adrenals. You don't want your blood sugar and hormones both going haywire at the same time. Eating low- to medium-glycemic foods can help reduce mood swings, lower anxiety, improve your energy levels and help with your weight-loss plan.

Choose your carbs cautiously! Aim to consume low- to medium-level carbohydrates.

Low Glycemic (55 or less)	Medium Glycemic (56-69)	High Glycemic (70+)
Bran cereals	Brown rice	French fries
Legumes	Oatmeal	White potatoes
High-fiber fruits (apple, plums, oranges, cherries) and vegetables (broccoli)	Rice cakes	Candy bars
	Rye bread	White rice
	Shredded wheat cereal	White-flour pasta
Plain yogurt	Whole-grain breads	Fruit juice with added sugar
Soy beverage	Whole-grain pasta	
Soy beans	Fruit juices without added sugar	Sugar-sweetened beverages
All-bran		
Skim Milk	Pineapple	Refined breakfast cereals
Sweet potato or yams	Banana	Watermelon
Hummus (chickpea salad dip)	Raisins	Dried dates
Pumpernickel bread	Popcorn	Sugary snacks
Sourdough wheat bread	Split peas	Soda crackers
	Couscous	Bagels, white
		Instant rice

Menopause Makeover Planner Entry:
Select healthy carbohydrate choices and enter them in your "shopping list" in Chapter 13.

MAKEOVER TIPS:

- Consume low- to medium-glycemic foods.
- Eat high fiber, complex carbs.
- If you consume a high-glycemic food, combine it with low GI food. For example, if you eat corn flakes for breakfast (high GI), add some strawberries (low GI) to make it a medium glycemic value.
- Include at least one low-glycemic choice for each meal.
- Substitute white bread with rye or oat-bran bread.
- Fruits and vegetables are great, healthy carb choices during the menopause transition.

FIBER IS OUR FRIEND

Fiber is the part of plants that cannot be digested. All fruits, grains, vegetables and legumes contain fiber. Fiber is usually found in the outer layer of the plant, and is considered a carbohydrate. When you eat fiber, it passes through your body virtually unchanged.

Benefits of fiber

* Helps keep your bowel movements regular and stools soft.
* Moves fat through your digestive system quicker--an added benefit in the battle against mid-section belly fat.
* Can help you lose weight.
* Leaves you feeling full longer.
* Keeps your blood sugar on an even keel.
* Can help transport bad cholesterol out of your body.
* Can help reduce the risk of certain diseases (heart disease, diabetes).

Fiber is broken down into two categories, insoluble and soluble. Insoluble fiber cannot be dissolved in water. Soluble fiber can dissolve in water.

SOURCES OF FIBER

Soluble

Apples	Strawberries	Blueberries	Pears	Apple pulp
Beans	Lentils	Rice bran	Oatmeal	
Nuts	Seeds	Oat bran	Peas	

Insoluble

Carrots	Cucumbers	Celery	Tomatoes	Cabbage
Zucchini	Whole-wheat	Brown rice	Barley	Brussels sprouts
Couscous	breads	Wheat bran	Rye	Cauliflower
	Whole-grain			Beets
	cereals			

Menopause Makeover Planner Entry:
Add your healthy fiber choices to your "shopping list" in Chapter 13.

One of the primary benefits of *soluble fiber* is it can lower blood cholesterol. And an excellent benefit of *insoluble fiber* is that it works as a laxative to move food along. You should consume 21 to 25 grams of fiber per day. Fiber is a wonderful part of your diet.

ALWAYS CARRY HEALTHY SNACKS ON THE ROAD.

MAKEOVER TIPS:

* Snack on raw vegetables and fruit when you get the munchies.
* Replace white pasta, breads and rice with whole-grain pasta, breads and rice.
* Incorporate a bowl of whole-grain cereal into your food plan for breakfast.

WATER

Two thirds of our body weight is water. Blood is 83 percent water, muscles 75 percent, bone 22 percent and the brain 74 percent. So water is obviously good for you. Without water you would dehydrate, and your vital organs would shutdown. Water is a necessity for life itself. Water is the most important molecule, second to oxygen, to live.

Benefits of drinking water:

* Keeps skin healthy and radiant.
* Water helps regulate body temperature.
* Water transports nutrients to your organs.
* Water removes waste.
* Water maintains overall health.

How much water do you need to consume?

There is no one water consumption formula that works for everyone. The Institute of Medicine advises that women consume 9 cups (2.2 liters) of total beverages per day.

YOUR PERSONAL WATER NEEDS DEPEND ON MANY FACTORS:

- For every 20 minutes of exercise you do each day, drink 8 ounces of water.
- Hot or humid weather can increase sweating, increasing your fluid retention.
- If you are ill, suffering from a fever, vomiting or diarrhea causing a loss of fluids, drink more water. If you are suffering from kidney, liver or adrenal disease, discuss your water intake with your doctor.
- If you drink alcohol, add an equal amount of water. For example, 6 ounces of wine should be matched with 6 ounces of water consumption.
- Bottom line: hydrate based on your needs.

On average, 80% of your body's water comes from drinking water and beverage sources, and 20% of water comes from food sources. Many women consume coffee, tea, and sodas, thinking it is a source for water. Although it is made mostly with water, nothing can replace the enormous benefits of pure water. Limit yourself to no more than two three-ounce cups of caffeine (coffee, tea, soda) per day. If you are on blood pressure medication such as diuretics, or have a history of heart problems or swelling in your legs, you may need to adjust your fluid intake, so discuss this with your health care provider!

MAKEOVER TIPS:

- Drink more water during exercise to replace water loss from sweating.
- If you don't like to drink water, enjoy fruits, which are high in water content.
- Drink sparkling water on ice with a twist of lemon.
- If you consume caffeinated drinks (coffee, tea, soda), alcohol drinks or salty foods drink more water to avoid dehydration.

LIMIT ALCOHOL

Too much alcohol can disrupt your sleep and trigger hot flashes. Lately there have been new reports claiming minimal red wine consumption is good for you. It can be, but no more than 6 ounces per day. Remember, red wine has calories, too.

SALT BEWARE

Just as we cannot live without water, we cannot live without salt. When we cry, our tears are salty. When we sweat, our perspiration is salty. Salt can cure, seal, clean, preserve, and act as an antiseptic. And salt is absolutely calorie-free.

So, what *is* salt? It is a dietary mineral and essential for human life. It is composed of sodium chloride. The body needs a certain amount of sodium to function properly. The average adult contains approximately 250 grams of salt (that is about four salt shakers' worth of salt). We lose salt through normal body functions, so it is important to consume a healthy amount of salt daily. Unlike water, consuming too much salt is not beneficial. If you eat too much salt, your body may retain water, causing weight gain, increased blood pressure and hypertension, which increases your risk of stroke and heart disease.

Benefits of salt

- Helps the body absorb potassium.
- Helps maintain the correct concentration of body fluids.
- It is an important part of transmitting electrical impulses in the nerves.
- Helps cells to absorb nutrients.
- The sodium in salt is needed to ensure our muscles and nerves work properly.
- The sodium in salt also helps maintain normal blood pressure.

The American Heart Association recommends less than 2,300 milligrams (one teaspoon) of salt per day. Almost all processed foods, junk food, chips, bacon, cheese, pickles, fast food, meat products, and breads have high levels of salt. Recent studies reveal that 77 percent of a person's salt intake is from processed foods. Throw in the salt we add to food during preparation and eating, and most people are over-consuming salt.

The Center for Science in the Public Interest claims excess salt is the single most harmful element in the food supply—even worse than saturated fat and trans fat, or food additives and pesticides! Salt is also a major cause of high blood pressure. During menopause, eliminating salt from your diet will help alleviate fluid retention. Do not add salt to your food and reduce your overall salt intake by eating fewer processed foods and being mindful of your salt intake.

REASONS TO QUIT

If you are a smoker, now is a good time to stop. Smoking has been linked with early menopause, and oftentimes with the appearance of wrinkles earlier in life. More than 178,000 women die each year from smoking-related diseases. It is not too late to quit smoking. There are chewing gums, prescriptions, patches and support groups to help you quit. If you smoke now is the time to quit.

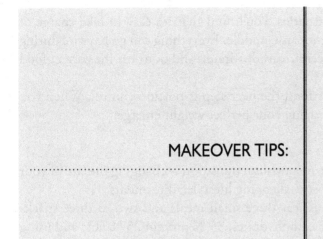

MAKEOVER TIPS:

- Don't add salt while cooking or at the table.
- Eat fresh foods, they do not have salt added.
- Season with herbs and spices instead of salt (lemon, garlic, paprika).
- Avoid processed foods (frozen meals, fast foods, convenience foods and many canned foods).
- Use soy sauce sparingly (created by soaking soy beans in salt).
- Avoid bacon, sausages, ham, cheese, pizzas and stock cubes.
- Avoid salted chips, nuts, crackers or other salty snacks.

THE MENOPAUSE MAKEOVER FOOD PYRAMID

There are no official government studies on what the correct eating ratios are for menopausal women. I had the task of exploring different ratios for myself. What I discovered was that I had to increase my protein intake, and decrease my high-glycemic carbohydrate intake. The answer is *The Menopause Makeover* food pyramid—the key to eating during menopause.

The Menopause Makeover Food Pyramid

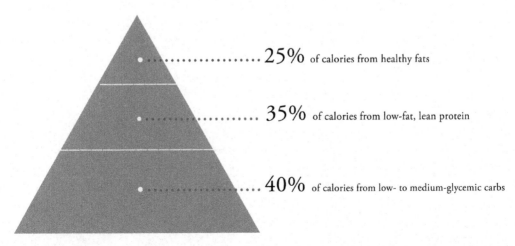

25% of calories from healthy fats

35% of calories from low-fat, lean protein

40% of calories from low- to medium-glycemic carbs

If you make this adjustment in your food ratios, you'll find that it's easy to take charge of your weight and keep from packing on the menopause middle. Everything can go haywire during menopause when you over-consume high-gylcemic carbohydrates, and don't eat the correct food ratios for your changing body.

Once you achieve the proper food proportions, the next step is portion control. When you combine these two elements, you will start noticing your perfect weight emerge!

PORTION CONTROL

One of the hardest adjustments during the menopausal transition is changing the size of your food portions. For me, this was one of the most challenging lifestyle adjustments.

During the menopause transition you must eat three small meals and two to three snacks every day, honoring the new food ratios (40 % carbohydrates, 35 % protein 25 % fats) and using these portions:

CORRECT FOOD PORTIONS

PROTEIN: size and thickness of your palm – 4 to 6 oz.

CARBOHYDRATES: size of your fist (wrist to knuckles) or tennis ball – 1 cup raw, ½ cup cooked, or medium size

FATS: size of your thumb

WATER: 6 to 8 8-ounce glasses

COFFEE: less than two cups per day

ALCOHOL: less than 6 oz per day

MAKEOVER TIPS	• Fill over a third of your plate with lean protein, and the rest with low glycemic carbohydrates, and sprinkle some healthy fat.
	• Purchase smaller plates. This strategy really helped me *think* I had a full plate of food.
	• When preparing your weekly food plan, each meal should follow the Menopause Makeover food pyramid

THE CALORIE COP, YOUR FRIENDLY PORTION CONTROL ENFORCEMENT

During your Menopause Makeover, you should count your calories daily. This will require some effort, but the pay-off is you will see first-hand whether or not you are overeating. Even overeating healthy foods can add weight. This exercise will help you learn to adjust your portion sizes. After tracking your calories for a couple of weeks, you'll start to notice if your eating habits and portion size are working in your favor. I discovered two weeks into my makeover that I was overeating a favorite snack, veggies and hummus. Hummus is a wonderful snack, but it is high in calories.

We will discuss calories more in Chapter 10, and then calculate your calorie intake in Chapter 11. Then you will apply this information in your daily food portion of your 12-Week Essential Planner.

THE THERMIC EFFECT OF FOOD, YOUR SECRET WEAPON

When you honor The Menopause Makeover Food Pyramid, you will be using the thermic effect of food to help burn that stubborn menopause belly fat. The thermic effect of food is the amount of energy it takes your body to digest food.

Thermic Effect for:
Proteins: About 30%
Carbohydrates: About 20%
Fats: About 3%

Your body is using more energy to digest protein, helping you speed up your metabolism. A higher metabolism is your secret weapon to weight loss and good health. Knowing what foods speed up your metabolism can help you lose weight, and burn that belly fat. We will calculate the thermic effect of food for your Menopause Makeover in Chapter 11.

SUPPLEMENTS

The best way to achieve nutritional health is by eating a diet rich in vitamins and minerals. Our bodies require more than 45 vitamins and minerals to maintain good health. Many of us do not consume a healthy diet, so there can be benefits to taking supplements. Supplements can have positive benefits during the menopausal transition. See the resources in the back of the book for a chart of dietary supplements.

Your body was designed to absorb nutrients from food sources. Consuming a healthy diet that includes natural food sources is the healthiest choice. Taking a daily multi-vitamin with minerals can be a good option as a supplement to a healthy diet. Discuss all supplement choices with your healthcare provider. Vitamins and minerals can affect your health if combined with certain drugs; and many medications deplete your body of essential nutrients.

If you have health concerns, such as kidney stones, high cholesterol, high blood pressure or heart disease, notify your doctor of any new supplements added to your daily plan. If you are taking high dosages of aspirin daily, consult your doctor before adjusting your supplements.

CALCIUM WITH VITAMIN D

During menopause it is advisable that you get enough calcium and vitamin D for bone health. The current recommendation for calcium is to get as much as possible in dietary form (yogurt, milk, dark leafy greens, fortified cereals, soybeans) because dietary calcium is easier to absorb.

Calcium plus vitamin D has been shown to reduce bone loss in healthy postmenopausal women, and also in postmenopausal women with substantial bone loss. If you cannot take in 500 to 1000 mg of calcium daily, then supplement with just one 500 mg tablet, taken with food, and separately from any other medications. There is scientific evidence that maintaining a healthy vitamin D level contributes to good health. You can purchase vitamin D3, 1000 IU, over the counter. Discuss calcium with vitamin D choices with your practitioner

---

Menopause Makeover Planner Entry:
Record daily supplements in your daily planner.

FEEDING THE NEW YOU

Making healthy food choices can change your life. Eating fast food and processed food, and overeating unhealthy foods, will only continue to contribute to a miserable menopause experience. Your food choices may be one of the most important changes you can make that will benefit you the rest of your life.

Once you start properly feeding the healthy girl hiding under a fat suit, your perfect weight will emerge. Many menopause symptoms may disappear, your emotional health and self-esteem may improve, too. Eating the proper foods in the correct amounts will help you achieve a healthy weight.

Making smart decisions regarding food for your 12-Week Menopause Makeover is often the most difficult part of managing menopause. If you reach for food for emotional support, now is the time to challenge yourself and conquer emotional issues. Remember, you can set yourself free with food!

KEEPING A DIARY AND CREATING A FOOD PLAN

Part of *The Menopause Makeover* plan is to keep a daily food diary and a weekly food plan. A daily food diary is a powerful tool for holding you accountable to your goals. Ladies who use a food diary lose almost twice the weight as those who do not. Your food diary will help identify areas that need improvement, so you can make necessary changes. Eating a healthy diet, maintaining a healthy weight, and exercising may reduce your risk of disease.

There are food plan templates in Chapter 13, the Essential Planner. Design your food plans weekly. Having a plan is important, so you can achieve your food goals.

Menopause Makeover Planner Entry:

Make food and menu choices before your start each week. Prepare a shopping list that honors that plan using the sample list in the Essential Planner. Review a sample food plan in Chapter 13 of the Essential Planner. Fill in the blank food plans with your weekly food choices, following your daily calorie intake.

MAKEOVER TIPS:

* Eat the correct combination of foods (35% protein, 40% carbs, 25% fat) at every meal.
* Always eat within an hour of waking up.
* Eat 3 meals, and 2-3 snacks per day.
* Don't let yourself get hungry; never let more than 4 hours go by without eating.
* Drink lots of water.
* Have no more than one glass of alcohol per day.
* Have no more than two cups of coffee per day.
* Get your daily calcium from dietary sources. Get plenty of sleep.
* Record everything you eat and drink in your 12-Week Planner.
* Do not salt food or prepare food with salt.
* Enjoy healthy snacks with plenty of filling fiber.
* Watch your portions when eating out and avoid simple carbs like the breadbasket. If the portion is too large, ask the waiter to take half and wrap it up for lunch the next day.
* Brown bag a healthy lunch to stick to your food plan. You will save money and calories!
* If you are having a bad food day, don't beat yourself up – just get back on the plan the next day.
* Reward yourself when you have success. Go shopping for a pair of sexy shoes, rather than treating yourself to ice cream.

MAKEOVER TAKE ACTION LIST

- Clear the kitchen of any foods not on your list of good proteins, carbohydrates and fats.
- Go to the grocery store with your shopping list of healthy foods, and purchase only foods listed on your food plan.
- If cooking for your family, start preparing meals following your plan. Making healthy food choices is good for the whole family.
- Start incorporating ways to cope with stress daily.
- If you are an emotional eater, identify the reason and confront it.
- Be honest when answering why you may be hiding under a fat suit. Discuss with a close friend. Getting outside input may help you answer this question.

IN YOUR ESSENTIAL PLANNER

- Record nutritional goals.
- Select your preferred healthy protein, fat, carbohydrate, and fiber choices and add to your shopping list.
- Tape a copy of The Menopause Makeover Food Pyramid to your refrigerator door
- Record all food intake daily in your 12-Week Planner.
- Prepare Food Plans each week using the sample in Chapter 13.
- Track your nutritional goals progress daily in your 12-Week Planner.

| Chapter 4 | Step Three: Exercise It Off
You Think Hot Flashes are Bad?
Now It's Time to BURN Baby BURN! |

I created my own version of the seven dwarfs to describe my menopausal body: saggy, droopy, baggy, lumpy, frumpy, flabby, and hefty! It wasn't enough to just eat healthfully, I wanted to look healthy, and that meant adding exercise to my lifestyle.

Waking up at the crack of dawn and stuffing myself into an out-of-date, neon colored exercise outfit, I'd dash out of the house, hiding under a big floppy hat, to begin power walking. Once I made a promise to feed and exercise my healthy self, I decided power walking would be the only exercise I had the strength to actually endure. After months of pigging out and feeling sorry for myself, I had lost my endurance, lung capacity, and muscle tone. Not to mention my joints were not accustomed to carrying around my extra weight. I was embarrassed about my body. There was no way I was going to a gym or yoga class with walls of mirrors where others could witness my mushy lumpy body trying to hide under a muumuu T-shirt.

With a spring in my power-walking step, assuming my commitment and good attitude were all it was going to take to get healthy again, I was huffing and puffing after just 15 minutes at a slow pace. My heart was pounding, and I was drenched with sweat.

My health was in serious jeopardy. How was I ever going to get my power back? It took two weeks, five days a week, to finally power-walk 15 minutes without feeling doomed. I thought exercise was supposed to feel invigorating. Yet all I felt was discouraged.

After building some endurance, I added time and increased my pace, as well as intensity — every day until I started seeing results. The endorphins were flowing again, and I felt happier. I could feel my strength coming back. Each week my fat suit slowly unzipped. There were days I dragged myself out of the house, dreading the workout. It was hard work. It took more than great effort. It took getting educated. I needed to understand my body and why it was failing me during menopause. I thought hot flashes were bad, but exercise was an uphill battle! After three months of exercise, I slipped back into my skinny jeans. Adding exercise to your daily schedule can increase the number of years you will live, it feels good, and it helps you look good.

We live in a society that supports and promotes youth. Youthful firm bodies are used to sell shampoo, clothes, cars, and beauty products. We hardly ever see a real-looking 50-year-old woman in a shampoo ad. Even the "older" models are attractive with unnaturally skinny bodies. It is discouraging to be slapped in the face with billboards, magazine ads, commercials, TV shows, and movies starring the young and beautiful. It can make it twice as difficult to think there is hope of getting back into shape, reclaiming your health and beauty.

The good news is that once you add exercise to your daily routine, you have taken an enormous step for your health. A regular exercise routine will help you fight the clock and will relieve a number of menopause symptoms, including depression, crankiness, joint aches, muscle tension, high blood pressure, fatigue, and anxiety as well as age-related concerns

This chapter will cover exercise information needed to make choices for your personal Menopause Makeover. You will have the tools necessary to design an exercise plan that fits into your lifestyle. If you want to feel good, look good, conquer many diseases, and age more gracefully, you must incorporate daily exercise. Without exercise, the quality of your survival declines and menopausal symptoms can increase. Who wants to be a menopausal blob of flab inviting age, and disease?

EXERCISE: YOUR FOUNTAIN OF YOUTH

Not only can daily exercise lower blood pressure and cholesterol, help you lose weight, slow or prevent osteoporosis, and reduce anxiety, but *not* exercising actually increases your risk of many preventable diseases, including heart disease, certain cancers, and type 2 diabetes.

Studies confirm that 20 to 30 minutes of exercise a day not only helps you live longer, but healthier. During exercise you breathe deeper, increasing the amount of oxygen in your bloodstream; your heart beats harder, increasing the blood flow to your lungs and muscles, and helping carry away waste products; and your body releases endorphins, the feel-good hormones. You can't get enough endorphins during menopause!

Tragically, knowing the benefits of exercise is not enough—you have to actually go out and do it. Most of us do not have the time or desire to include exercise in our daily regime, but the benefits are worth the effort. As we age – losing muscle mass and a youthful metabolism – menopause throws in a whole new set of challenges. During "the change" it may seem as if every day a new physical ailment crops up – night sweats, muscle aches, or moodiness. Exercise can help with all of this.

If you are a baby boomer determined not to look mortality in the face, then exercise can be your fountain of youth.

BENEFITS OF EXERCISE

Lowers blood pressure	Can enhance sexual pleasure
Increases bone density	Lowers risk of Type-2 Diabetes
Increases strength	Increases general mobility
Lowers blood sugar	Burns calories
Strengthens your heart	Helps you feel healthier and happier
Strengthens lungs	Strengthens joints and ligaments
Increases your stamina	Strengthens your immune system
Reduces anxiety and stress	Lowers risk of some cancers
Improves self-esteem	Lowers risk of heart disease
Increases your metabolism	Builds healthy muscles, bones and joints
Improves digestive function	Increases good cholesterol and decreases bad cholesterol

HEART HEALTH

One of the greatest exercise benefits is having a healthy heart. The leading killer of American women is heart attack. More than five times as many women die of heart attacks than from breast cancer. Menopause is associated with an increased risk of heart disease, making exercise that much more important.

What does menopause have to do with heart health?

After menopause, your risk for cardiovascular disease and high blood pressure significantly increases. At this time, there is still controversy, suggesting estrogen may provide cardioprotective benefits of estrogen. Throw in factors such as aging, a family history of heart disease, smoking, excessive alcohol consumption, a poor diet with too much salt intake, obesity, and stress, and your risk of suffering from heart disease and high blood pressure increases.

What is blood pressure?

Over 39 million women have high blood pressure. Blood pressure is the force of blood against your artery walls. When you heart pumps blood out, it is called *systolic* pressure. When your heart is at rest between the beats, it is called *diastolic* pressure. When your doctor takes a blood pressure reading the top or first number is the systolic pressure, and the bottom or second number is the diastolic pressure. Normal blood pressure is less than 130/90.

High blood pressure is known as the silent killer because there are no symptoms and yet it can increase your risk of stroke, heart failure, kidney failure or heart attack. Age and genetics are the most common causes for high blood pressure. Weight gain and fluid retention can also contribute.

There's good news, exercise can lower your blood pressure. If you suffer from high blood pressure, add exercise to your daily routine, even if you are on blood pressure medication. Lifestyle changes may delay or reduce your risk of heart disease and high blood pressure. Regular exercise will build a stronger heart pumping more blood with less effort, and that equals less pressure on your arteries. Committing to daily exercise may help you avoid blood pressure medications all together. Monitor your blood pressure daily and discuss strategies to manage high blood pressure with your doctor.

START EXERCISING YOUR BODY... YOUR HEART WILL LOVE YOU FOR IT!

BONE HEALTH

Weight-bearing and resistance exercises are the only exercises that can actually enhance bone growth and stop bone loss. When you do weight-bearing or resistance exercises, you force your muscles to work against gravity. The exercise causes your muscles to contract against the bone. Bone is living tissue, and this contraction stimulates new bone growth, so that your bones actually grow stronger and denser.

Weight-bearing and resistance exercises also make it possible for bones to absorb more calcium. After the age of 30, women begin to lose bone mass and the risk of osteoporosis increases with menopause. Do not be a victim of poor bone health. Most of us want a tight butt and firm tummy; but without strong bones, both are impossible. You need healthy bones to carry your body around the rest of your life. There is no cure for osteoporosis, but it is treatable. Make a commitment to your bone health and exercise!

WEIGHT-BEARING EXERCISES

Jogging	Power walking	Hiking
Step aerobics	Tennis	Jumping
Dancing	Climbing stairs	

RESISTANCE/STRENGTHENING EXERCISES

Weight-lifting	Free weights	Weight machines
Elastic tubing	Push-ups	

If You Have Osteoporosis

If you have a diagnosis of osteoporosis, consult with your health-care provider before starting a new exercise program. Your doctor might recommend low-impact exercises, like walking or swimming laps, and may also advise you against exercise that involve twisting, reaching or bending the spine

INCREASED METABOLISM

One of the greatest benefits of exercise is that it can increase your metabolism. Your muscles burn 10 to 12 calories per pound, per 24-hour period, even while you are sleeping. During menopause you lose muscle mass, so on top of weight gain, your metabolism slows.

The good news is that muscle burns more calories than fat, and increases your metabolism. Now is the time to start toning your muscles so you can raise your metabolism. Now is the time to start toning your muscles so you can raise your metabolism.

FOCUS ON BEING HEALTHY.

THE MENOPAUSE MAKEOVER EXERCISE FORMULA

Now you know the great things exercise can do for your body. So, how do you get started? First you need to understand the different types of exercises you can do.

THREE TYPES OF EXERCISE

There are three ways to exercise:

1. **Flexibility Exercises** reduces the risk of exercise related injuries, maintains joint range of motion, so you can enjoy both cardiovascular, and strength training activities.

2. **Strength Training** using weight bearing or resistance exercises can strengthen muscles burning fat, increasing lean muscle mass, boosting metabolism, and strengthening bones.

3. **Cardiovascular Exercise** at your target heart rate can speed up metabolism and burn calories.

Five to six days a week you will do 5 minutes to 10 minutes of stretching to maintain flex-ibility. Then you will add twenty to thirty minutes of cardio, at your target heart rate, for endurance and overall health. Two to three times a week, add strength training to build muscle tone. All you have to do is exercise 40 minutes most days of the week. That equals one TV show, the time to pack the kids' lunches (teach them how to make lunch), time to pick up the house in the morning (ask your partner to help, so you can exercise), or time on the phone with a friend (chat while you are power walking). Making time for exercise is possible. Consider exercise a Menopause Makeover prescription!

THE MENOPAUSE MAKEOVER EXERCISE FORMULA:

| **Flexibility Exercises 5 – 10 minutes most days of the week** | **+ Strength Training 2 – 3 days a week** | **+ Cardiovascular 20 - 30 minutes most days of the week** | **= Good Fitness!** |

FLEXIBILITY EXERCISES

Many of us rush into exercise routines without making time for proper stretching. Flexible muscles can reduce the chances of injury. As we age, our tendons and ligaments begin to stiffen, limiting our range of motion and making it painful to move. Stretching can stimulate the production of lubricants between the connective tissue fibers, reversing some of these effects of aging.

BENEFITS OF STRETCHING

- Reduces muscle tension.
- Increases body coordination.
- Keeps muscles supple.
- Does not cause pain when done correctly.
- Warms up muscles.
- Can reduce stress, feels relaxing.
- Feels good.
- Reduces risk of exercise-related injuries.
- Easy to learn.

- Maintains joint range of motion.
- You can stretch anywhere.
- Can prevent other injuries.
- Enhances flexibility.
- Enhances overall body image.
- You can stretch anytime.
- Increases body temperature and heart rate.
- Develops body awareness.
- Increases ability to achieve physical relaxation.

Always warm up a few minutes before stretching. You can turn the heat up, take a hot shower, walk around, march in place – just don't start stretching with tense muscles. Get your blood moving first. Raising your blood temperature prior to stretching will allow you to do your stretching routine with reduced risk of injury. Warm muscles are more pliable than cold ones.

MAKEOVER TIPS:

- Stretch slowly.
- Commit yourself to proper technique.
- Breathe out when at the maximum part of stretch.
- Do not bounce.
- Breathe naturally, but do not hold your breath.
- Try to stretch a little farther on each stretch, during the exhale.
- Hold a stretch 10-15 seconds if you are a beginner, and work your way up to 30 seconds. per stretch as your muscles become more flexible.

When you first start, go slowly, focusing on proper technique.

STRENGTH TRAINING

The best way to strengthen muscles is to add resistance. When you fatigue a muscle or muscle group, lactic acids build up, causing a burning sensation. This is a wake-up call to those unused muscles to start working again. Your body will begin to synthesize new tissue to meet the demands you are putting on that muscle. Toning up a muscle requires progressive muscle resistance. Introducing more weight than the muscle can handle will help it grow stronger. Unlike cardio, where you work your body for a longer period of time, strength training puts stress on the muscle for a shorter period of time but at a higher intensity. Aging during the menopause transition results in lean muscle mass loss; strength training will restore your muscle tissue. Toning those flabby arms, jiggly belly and wiggly booty will not only give you added strength, but your self-esteem will skyrocket, too!

Benefits of strength training
- Builds muscle.
- Burns calories, raises metabolism.
- Promotes bone health.
- Increases endurance and strength.
- Improves flexibility and coordination.
- Improves self-esteem.

Once you add strength training to your exercise routine you will witness how quickly your body adapts: you'll see changes before you know it.

Common strength equipment: weight machines (gym or home gym models), free weights (dumbbells and barbells), resistance bands (elastic tubing with handles and elastic bands), or using your body weight (pull-ups and push-ups).

Exercise the larger muscles first, so you do not exhaust the smaller muscle groups that are needed to exercise the larger muscles. Rest a day between each group.

MAJOR MUSCLE GROUPS

Upper Body

CHEST: Pectorals, known as pecs

SHOULDERS: Deltoids, known as delts, rotator cuff

BACK: Trapezius and latissimus dorsi, known as traps and lats

LOWER BACK: erector spinae

ARMS: biceps, triceps, forearm

ABDOMINALS: rectus abdominis, known as abs,

OBILQUES AND WAIST: internal and external obliques

Lower body

OUTER THIGHS: hip abuductors

INNER THIGHS: leg adductors

BUTTOX: gluteus maximus, known as glutes

QUADRICEPS: known as quads

HAMSTRINGS: known as hams

SHINS: tibialis anterior

CALVES: gastrocnemius and soleus

CREATING A STRENGTH-TRAINING ROUTINE

An easy way to organize your strength training routine is to divide the upper and lower body (abs included in the lower body routine) every other day.

SAMPLE STRENGTH TRAINING ROUTINE

Monday	Upper body (back, chest, shoulders, triceps, biceps)
Tuesday	Rest
Wednesday	Lower body (glutes, quads, hams, calves, abs)
Thursday	Rest
Friday	Upper body (back, chest, shoulders, triceps, biceps)
Saturday	Rest
Sunday	Rest

CREATING A STRENGTH-TRAINING FORMULA

Now all you need to do is put it all together into a series of *reps* and *sets*. A *rep* is a repetition of the same resistance exercise. A *set* is the chosen number of repetitions of that resistance exercise in a row. Rest 30 to 90 seconds between each set. If you are a beginner start with a 90 second rest between sets.

COMMON STRENGTH TRAINING FORMULAS

Beginner	Intermediate	Advanced
1 set, 10 reps	2-3 sets, 10-12 reps	3 set, 12-15 reps

For your abs, do 10 to 25 reps at your appropriate "set" level

When your workout becomes easy, add weight and change up your routines to keep it interesting and to stimulate the muscles.

MAKEOVER TIPS:

1. Don't hold your breath.
2. Hold dumbbell in the center of the handle, except for the overhead extensions.
3. Choose weights that are heavy enough to get through the scheduled number of reps. If the weight is not heavy enough, you will not stress the muscle enough to rebuild it.
4. Rest 30-90 seconds between sets.
5. Breathe in through your nose and out through your mouth. Breathe with full inhalations and exhalations. Exhale when your muscles are tightening.
6. If you want a cardio workout while strength training, do not rest between sets.
7. Wear comfy clothes that breathe, not too baggy and not too tight.

CARDIOVASCULAR EXERCISE

Once you select an enjoyable cardio activity that fits into your lifestyle, make a commitment to do it most days a week.

Benefits of cardiovascular activity

* Relieves stress.
* Improves heart function.
* Reduces risk of heart disease.
* Improves blood cholesterol and tri-glyceride levels.
* Reduces risk of osteoporosis.
* Improves muscle tone.
* Increases production of endorphins.
* Reduces risk of diabetes.
* Helps with weight management.
* Increases lung capacity.
* Helps you sleep better.
* Boosts mood.

MAKEOVER TIPS:

* Discuss your program with your doctor.
* Schedule cardio workouts on your calendar.
* Aim to do at least 20-30 continuous minutes most days of the week.
* Make sure you are using good gear or equipment.

TOP 10 CARDIO EXERCISES

Calories burned in 30 minutes, for a 145-pound woman

Step Aerobics	400 calories	Cross-Country Skiing	330 calories
Bicycling	250-500 calories	Running	300 calories
Swimming	400 calories	Elliptical Machine	300 calories
Playing racquetball	400 calories	Rowing	300 calories
Rock Climbing	380 calories	Walking	180 calories

If you are jogging or power walking, owning a good pair of shoes is important to avoid injury. Also, consider incorporating music, reading or watching TV during your training, so you don't get bored. Wrangle a friend and have fun chatting during your session. Don't forget to mix it up. If you are working out at the gym, switch between the elliptical cross-trainer and the treadmill. If you power walk in your neighborhood, try hiking or biking with a friend for variety.

SAMPLE WORKOUT SCHEDULE

Monday	Warm-up/stretch, strength training, cardio
Tuesday	Warm-up/stretch, cardio
Wednesday	Warm-up/stretch, strength training, cardio
Thursday	Warm-up/stretch, cardio
Friday	Warm-up/stretch, strength training, cardio
Saturday	Warm-up/stretch, cardio
Sunday	REST

WHEN TO EXERCISE AND FOR HOW LONG

You can exercise any time of the day. Many people prefer to do it first thing in the morning, and start the day fresh. Others like to exercise at the end of their day to release tension. And others split up their exercise routines between morning and evening to work it into their busy schedules. The days you incorporate strength training, I recommend two sessions if you need to break up your routine. Do your stretches and strength training in the morning, and 20 to 30 minutes of cardio later in the day, or vice versa. If you plan to do this, remember to warm-up a few minutes before your cardio segment.

Do not eat a heavy meal just before exercising. Consume something light, like an apple for energy before your exercise routine. Eat a balanced meal within two hours of completing your exercise regime.

BURNING CALORIES

Every time I clean and vacuum the house, I feel good knowing my house looks great, and I just zapped a couple hundred calories. That equals a glass of red wine or small yummy dessert. See where your brain can go when you have the information? You may ask, "If it is all about calories, why don't I just decrease my food intake and who needs exercise?" Do you cut food calories? Or increase exercise?

The *Journal of Clinical Endocrinology & Metabolism*, and the USDA confirm weight loss is about the calories. The more you burn baby burn, the more weight you will lose. In fact, consuming 500 fewer calories per day (just add a power walk and cut out a bagel) and you will lose a pound a week. I have found it easier to negotiate my day knowing I can use both food and exercise calories to meet my goals. Plus, exercise tones your muscles, and increases your heart and breathing rates – equaling good health with a healthy self-esteem. Cutting only food calories can be challenging, but exercise and physical activity is a wonderful tool to burn extra calories.

This lifestyle change is about balance, making a daily commitment to your health. Have a plan every day. Think about what you will be eating and when you'll get your workout in. If you have time, squeeze in a fun physical activity, like a walk during lunch. Even if you don't want to lose weight, exercise will help you maintain a healthy weight and lifestyle.

I discovered early in my quest for good health during menopause that not all women burn the exact amount of calories per activity. It depends on your weight and the intensity level you are moving at.

Do not compare yourself, or your exercise results, with someone else. Your goals and your results are unique only to you.

CALORIES BURNED PER HOUR

Circle 3 Activities That You Can Do For Your Menopause Makeover

SELECT YOUR WEIGHT CATEGORY	130 LB	155 LB	190 LB
Aerobics, general	354	422	518
Bicycling, less than 10mph, leisure	236	281	345
Bicycling, stationary—moderate effort	413	493	604
Bowling	177	211	259
Canoeing, rowing—moderate effort	413	493	604
Cleaning house—general	207	246	302
Dancing—general	266	317	388
Exercise equipment, cardio	354	422	518
Gardening	295	352	431
Golfing, general	236	281	345
Health club excercise—general	325	387	474
Hiking, cross-country	354	422	518
Horse grooming	354	422	518
Horse riding—general	236	281	345
Horse riding—trotting	382	457	561
Jogging—general	413	493	604
Kayaking	295	352	431
Rope jumping—moderate	590	704	863
Rowing, stationary—moderate effort	413	493	604
Running, 5 mph (12-min. mile)	472	563	690
Running, 5.2 mph (11.5-min. mile)	531	633	776
Running, 6 mph (10-min. mile)	590	704	863

SELECT YOUR WEIGHT CATEGORY	130 LB	155 LB	190 LB
Running, 6.7 mph (9-min. mile)	648	774	949
Running—general	472	563	690
Running—in place	472	563	690
Running up stairs	885	056	1294
Sailing, boat/board, windsurfing	177	211	259
Skating, ice—general	413	493	604
Skating, roller	413	493	604
Skiing, cross-country—moderate effort	472	563	690
Skiing, snow—general	413	493	604
Snowshoeing	472	563	690
Softball or baseball, fast or slow pitch	295	352	431
Stretching, hatha yoga	236	281	345
Surfing, body or board	177	211	259
Swimming laps, freestyle	472	563	690
Swimming, leisurely—general	354	422	518
Swimming, treading water—moderate	236	281	345
Table tennis	236	281	345
Tai chi	236	281	345
Teaching aerobics class	354	422	518
Tennis—doubles	354	422	518
Tennis—general	413	493	604
Tennis—singles	472	563	690

SELECT YOUR WEIGHT CATEGORY	130 LB	155 LB	190 LB
Volleyball—beach	472	563	690
Walking, 2.0 mph—slow pace	148	176	216
Walking, 3.0 mph—moderate pace	207	(246)	302
Walking, 3.5 mph—uphill	354	422	518
Walking, 4.0 mph—very brisk pace	236	281	345
Walking—grass track	295	352	431
Walking—upstairs	472	563	690
Water aerobics, water calisthenics	236	281	345
Waterskiing	354	422	518
Water volleyball	177	211	259
Weight lifting/body building vigorous	354	422	518
Weight lifting—light or moderate effort	177	211	259

Source: Department of Health and Family Services, State of Wisconsin.

Calories Burned Per Hour. 2005.

Available at: https://www.dhs.wisconsin.gov/publications/p4/p40109.pdf

The good news is that you burn calories all day during normal activities, too. But don't think this is an excuse to skip the gym!

DAILY ACTIVITIES WITH CALORIES BURNED PER HOUR

Sleeping	55	Knitting	85	Driving	110
Eating	85	Sitting	85	Office Work	140
Sewing	85	Standing	100	Housework	150

FINDING YOUR TARGET HEART RATE

How do you know if you are working hard enough to reap the benefits? One of the easiest ways to check your intensity is to monitor your heart rate. The target heart rate (THR) is your pulse rate per minute. When you train within your THR, you strengthen the cardiovascular system by exercising the heart, and increasing blood and oxygen flow to your body tissue. Your target heart rate is calculated at 60 to 80 percent of your maximum heart rate (MHR).

If you are a beginner, calculate the formula at 60 percent. When your routine becomes easy for you, then move up to 70 percent, then 80 percent as you get stronger.

If you are not using a cardio exercise machine with a heart rate monitor, you can purchase a heart rate monitor from $25.00 to $350.00. You can also take your pulse during exercising. Lightly place your two middle fingers on your throat at the jugular vein or you on your wrist over your pulse. Count your heartbeat for six seconds, and add a zero to that number.

The "talk test" is another good way to determine the intensity of your workout. If you can talk but are a little winded, then you are in your target zone. If you are completely winded and can barely talk, slow down. If chatting is too easy, step it up a notch (the cardio, not the chatting, that is). Always discuss your exercise choices with your doctor.

AVOIDING INJURIES

I was excited about starting a new exercise routine for my Menopause Makeover, so I jumped in with full effort, think-ing my body was still 20 years old. The first yoga class I took, I injured my rotator cuff (shoulder injury) doing Down Dog pose with too much energy for too long without the strength to support it. I visited the doctor, he injected cortisone, it healed, and then I went back to yoga class only to injure my lumbar 4/5 discs on a spinal twist.

HOW TO CALCULATE YOUR TARGET HEART RATE ZONE

Step #1:
Calculate your Maximum Heart Rate (upper limit of what your heart can handle during your workout)

220 – your age = MHR

Example for a 49-year-old woman: 220 – 49 = 171 MHR

Step #2:
Calculate your Target Heart Rate

**MHR x .60 = _____
(low-end range)**

**MHR x .70 = _____
(middle range)**

**MHR x .80 = _____
(high range)**

Example for a 49-year-old woman:
Her low-end range (60%)
171 x .60 = 102.6
Her middle range (70%)
171 x .70 = 119.7
Her high range (80%)
171 x .80 = 136.8

This 49-year-old's target heart rate is between 102.6 and 136.8 beats per minute.

First, with aging, ligaments and tendons are not as pliable. Second, my brain was acting like it was a 20-year-old not a 50-year-old. When you start the 12-Week Menopause Makeover Exercise Plan, start out slow and easy. Better to prevent an injury from the start. If you have history with an injury, such as knee or back issues, respect your injury. Do not overdo. Speak to your health-care practitioner before starting a new exercise plan. Whether you suffer from a torn ligament, muscles strain or joint concerns, make sure your daily exercise does not strain an existing injury. Always allow your injury to heal before putting stress on it again through exercise. You do not want an injury to turn into a permanent health concern.

MAKEOVER TIPS:

- If it hurts, don't use it.
- Warm-up and stretch before you begin any workout.
- Better to prevent an injury than to have to recover from one.
- If you are suffering from an injury, avoid all activity involving that body part or area.
- Do not over-train, go slowly focusing on proper form.
- Strengthen all your muscle groups, so your body is well balanced.
- If you have swelling, or severe pain, you may have an injury and should visit your doctor. For acute swelling, ice for 15-20 minutes, elevate and rest.
- Respect your body.

CHECK YOUR POSTURE

You can look pounds thinner and more confident with good posture. When you exercise, practice good posture. You know you have good posture when you can draw a straight line from your ear, through your shoulder, hip, and knee.

Sucking in your tummy and tucking your tush on a regular basis will help strengthen your muscles, and improve your appearance and mood. When you walk, stand, sit, and lie down, practice good posture. Once you begin your regular workout routine, having good posture will become automatic. Good posture will help prevent injuries during exercise, and you can look thinner and feel more confident.

STAYING MOTIVATED AND SETTING GOALS

One of the hardest commitments to make during your menopause transition is including exercise into your daily routine. It is so much easier to sit on the couch, and watch a movie enjoying a pint of ice cream. Trust me: You will feel better adding exercise to your life. Your self-esteem will improve, your clothes will fit better, you will have added strength, and you will add years to your life.

Tips on how to make exercise a habit for life!

1. Choose 5 activities you like that you can incorporate into your lifestyle. Anything from dancing, to power walking with the girls, to walking the dog, stair climbing, or window cleaning.

2. Set realistic goals.

3. Record all physical activity in your 12-Week Menopause Makeover Planner.

4. Mix it up! This ensures your body does not get used to the same activity and you no longer reap the benefits; and avoid boredom at all costs.

5. Schedule exercise in your 12-Week Menopause Makeover Planner.

6. If you are a procrastinator, and need motivation to get moving, attend scheduled classes.

7. Exercise at the same time every day, so it becomes part of your daily lifestyle.

8. Buy a cute exercise outfit, so you feel great working out.

9. Put together a music play-list on your iPod with upbeat tunes – motivating music goes a long way.

10. Watch your favorite TV shows while working out at the gym or on your home machine.

11. If you only have 15-20 minutes, use the time for strength training or a cardio session. Twenty minutes is better than no activity.

12. If you work out at home, create a space you like devoted to exercising.

13. Get an exercise buddy; socialize and burn calories together.

14. Exercise for a charity. Raise money for breast cancer; start training for Avon's 39-mile two-day benefit to raise money for breast cancer research. A good cause is a great motivator!

15. Reward yourself when you see results. Enjoy a day of shopping or pamper yourself with a spa day.

IF YOUR SCHEDULE IS TOO BUSY FOR EXERCISE, WAKE UP HALF HOUR EARLIER.

FIND THE RIGHT EXERCISE FOR YOU

If you are a person who needs a coach or leader, has energy in the afternoon, likes being social, prefers being indoors and isn't competitive, then joining a gym or taking a class (yoga, dancing) may be a good way to incorporate exercise into your lifestyle. Or get a group of friends together and alternate homes for a neighborhood power walk, and do your stretching and strength training together.

If you like the outdoors, do not need leadership, feel energized in the morning, and prefer having some alone time, then you may benefit from a morning power walk or hike combined with your stretching and strength training.

Honor yourself. Incorporating exercise into your lifestyle is a big commitment. You will need all odds in your favor.

Quiz | What type of exercise person are you?

1. Would prefer to have a coach tell you what to do, or do you like to be your own boss?

2. What time of day do you feel most energized? Morning? Afternoon? Evening?

3. Do you like to exercise with friends or solo?

4. Could you set up an area in your home to exercise? Or do you prefer to go to a gym or classroom?

5. Do you need a cheerleader to encourage you? Or do you have good motivation on your own?

6. Are you competitive with others in a class situation?

7. Do you like to exercise? If not, find a support team and organized exercise activities.

8. Would you prefer to get exercise through other activities like dancing or hiking?

9. Are you an indoor or outdoor person?

10. If you make a commitment to yourself, will you honor it?

HOW HEALTHY ARE YOU?

One of the best ways to motivate yourself is to set goals for improvement. Walking is a wonderful gauge to test your overall aerobic health. Take this test and find out how healthy you are. You can take this quiz using a treadmill with computerized distance and time settings, or mark off the distance in your neighborhood by driving (note the odometer reading at each mile) and time it yourself when walking.

ONE-MILE WALK FITNESS TEST

Record how long it takes you to walk one mile, then use these guidelines to rate your fitness level:

Fitness Level	Time
Fantastic	less than 11:44
Really great	11:45-13:11
Above average	13:10-14:34
Average	14:35-16:04
Not so good	16:05-17:29
Poor	more than 17:30

A brisk walk, 3.5 to 4.5 miles an hour, has cardiovascular benefits. After you determine your quiz results, you will be able to set goals to improve your health through exercise. When I launched a daily exercise routine, I was walking a 17:45-minute mile – a poor health grade! Six months later, I was walking a 14-minute mile. Just do it, your body will thank you. Now I power through a 13-minute mile with ease. My new goal is the 11:30 minute mile.

WHEN EXERCISING BECOMES A DRAG, ASK A BUDDY TO JOIN YOU.

CREATE YOUR OWN HOME GYM

Having a few exercise supplies at your home can increase your odds of incorporating exercise into your lifestyle. Find an area in your home designated for your workouts. I made a workout area in front of my bedroom mirror. I keep my exercise mat, dumbbells, and chair next to the mirror. THis equipment can be used for stretching, weight lifting with dumbbells and cardiovas-cular routines. THe exercise enthusiast may choose to purchase a home gym and cardiovascular machine (treadmill, elliptical).

MENOPAUSE MAKEOVER HOME GYM SUPPLIES

Full-length mirror	Yoga/exercise mat	Chair
Dumbbells	Heart rate monitor	Towels
Pedometer	Appropriate shoes	

CREATE A SUPPORT TEAM

Working out with friends is a wonderful way to socialize while reaping the benefits of exercise. Working out with a friend is a fun way to honor your commitment to exercise. Plus, having a gym buddy is great motivation to stick to your exercise routine.

NO MORE EXCUSES

Are you struggling or resisting the exercise challenge? "I don't have time," was my biggest reason to not exercise. Then I moved to a new city when I got married, and my explanation became "the gym is too far." Once I decided to power walk, because the gym was 20 minutes away, my new excuse became, "it is not safe to walk at night." Most of us have some pretty good excuses for not including exercise in our lifestyle.

MAKEOVER TIPS:

- Schedule workouts with friends in advance.
- Set goals with friends, enjoy a little competition with a tempting reward for success (that all can enjoy).
- Join a walking club.
- Take classes at your gym.
- Locate a nightclub that gives free dance classes and book that evening with a group of friends with similar dance interests.
- Combine exercise with other activities (create a dog-walking group, for instance).

WHAT'S YOUR EXCUSE NOT TO EXERCISE?

Make a check next to your favorite excuses—and next time you go to use one, don't!

CHECKLIST

Your Favorite Excuses

☐ Find exercise boring
☐ Do not have time to exercise
☐ Lack motivation and time management skills
☐ No confidence in your body
☐ Fear of being injured
☐ Exercise is an inconvenience
☐ Lack of support or encouragement
☐ No exercise location
☐ Were you the kid people made fun of during gym class?

What is the solution to your excuse not to exercise?

How can you create a positive remedy for your resistance to exercising?

EXERCISE CAN BE FUN AND SOCIAL. FOCUS ON DOING ACTIVITIES YOU ENJOY, INCLUDE FRIENDS, AND YOU HAVE A FORMULA FOR SUCCESS.

EXERCISE THE NEW YOU

Maximizing your workout will not only improve your overall health, it will give you a head start on battling menopausal weight gain, depression and saggy muscles. Exercise can also help deal with uncomfortable menopause symptoms, like hot flashes, anxiety, joint pain, and sleep disturbances. Plus, it reduces your risk of heart disease and osteoporosis!

REMEMBER:

What you think, you become
Having support is a powerful tool
Positive thinking goes a long way
Have one good laugh session a day
Reward yourself when you see progress

MAKEOVER TIPS

- Record your daily activity in your 12-Week Planner.
- Have a small snack 15-30 minutes before your workout (apple, yogurt, low-fat cottage cheese).
- Drink water during your exercise routine.
- Find small ways to burn calories during the day: take the stairs instead of the elevator, park your car at the far side of the mall parking lot, or stretch while you watch TV.
- Always plan your week in advance and schedule your workouts. If your schedule clears, throw in some stretches, cardio or strengthening exercises.
- Do not over-train – take it slow and easy, yet get a good workout.
- Variety is the spice of life – try new routines and activities, add friends, get a new playlist.
- Challenge yourself with intensity levels, times and new activities.

MAKEOVER TAKE ACTION LIST

- Prepare an area of your house to build your home gym, or join a local gym.
- Work out most days of the week.
- Always warm up for a few minutes.
- Practice good posture.
- Record all exercise goals on page 189.
- Record your Target Heart Rate.
- If you have high blood pressure, or cholesterol issues, record your levels.

IN YOUR ESSENTIAL PLANNER

- Record your selected workout routine in the monthly planner.
- Record daily workouts in your 12-Week Plan.
- List your workout buddies on page 209.
- Track exercise progress in Your Weekly Progress report.

Chapter 5

Step Four: Mirror, Mirror on the Wall, Is That Me?
Customizing Your Beauty Routine

I have stopped complaining about my blurry vision. For years, I looked in the mirror and saw someone in her early thirties. Of course, I wasn't wearing my reading glasses, so my out-of-focus vision was a blessing in disguise. After months of hearing me complain about my vision while I was applying makeup, a friend suggested I purchase a 5X-magnifying mirror. This solution was disastrous! Seeing myself in focus was horrifying. I looked like my mother! No offense, Mom. When did I get fine lines around my eyes? And those frown lines were now permanent fixtures hanging from my sagging cheeks and jowls.

The ugly truth is that menopause was taking its toll on my skin. The skin on my face was changing drastically; the skin on my arms looked like wrinkled dessert crêpes; the skin around my belly resembled a squashed donut; and the skin that supported my tush recently deflated, leaving a droopy booty. And, as if aging skin weren't bad enough, one morning I woke up to find a long black hair on my forehead. "It must be from my makeup brush!" When I went to brush it off, it remained attached. The one-inch black hair had sprung up overnight. A tweeze job followed by a stiff cup of coffee was the only solution.

With aging skin, declining vision, stray hairs, and a changing figure, feeling in control of your beauty may seem impossible.

Having worked with 40-something celebrities and their beauty teams during my television career, I realized I had some beauty secrets that needed dusting off. Years ago, a makeup artist confessed to me that her celebrity had a beauty secret that kept her skin gorgeous: weekly exfoliation. Years later, a costume designer quietly mentioned that his star looked ten pounds thinner because he had lowered her belt line. One of my greatest beauty discoveries happened when I entered the dressing room of a huge celebrity as she was having her microphone discreetly wired under her outfit. As the female sound person had the celebrity's dress pulled up to tape wires underneath, I sighted this beautiful over-50 star's toning undergarment (yep, a full-body girdle) from her bra to her thighs. When she caught me staring at her girdled body, she smiled and said, "One day you will need one too!" And she was right!

After months of serious exercise, my tummy was still a bowl of Jell-O – it was smaller, but loose and flabby. I purchased a sexy body-slimming suit with a built-in bra (inspired by that very wise movie star), and voila! My perky boobs and booty returned. If you are wondering who that movie star was…I will go to my grave with her name, but not her beauty secrets!

When you have a few beauty and styling tips in your arsenal, your 5X-magnifying mirror can be your friend. And don't be afraid to hang up the full-length mirror again!

This Chapter is packed with simple beauty and style tips, from skincare tips to monthly teeth whitening. You will enter beauty and style appointments in the month-at-a-glance calendar, so you can accomplish beauty goals during your menopause makeover.

HELP, I'M TURNING INTO MY MOTHER!

A few years ago, while on a waterskiing trip, I was bending over the outboard motor at the back of the powerboat tossing a water ski to a friend in the water. The boat driver called out, "Staness, toss out just one ski." As I turned to hear his command I could see a lumpy flabby butt in his rearview mirror. I thought, "My mom is not on this boa, so whose butt is that? She doesn't have the same swimsuit as I do." To my horror, it was *my* butt. I was in my forties, and I thought my booty was still sexy. My butt was now *my mother's butt*. Was I aging like my mother? My mother was starting to appear in my life everywhere. I started dressing like her to hide my ever-growing midsection and droopy butt. I noticed sagging skin under my chin, and some facial peach fuzz, just like Mom!

WHY IS MY SKIN WRINKLING AND SAGGING?

Thanks to aging and fluctuating hormones, I was quickly becoming my mother. Fortunately, I have a beautiful mother, but nothing was going to stop the inevitable--age and menopause.

During menopause we really start seeing the effects of aging. Your skin is supported by collagen and elastin fibers, which is why your skin looked so soft and contoured to your face before menopause. Throw in the loss of collagen, elastin and hyaluronic acid that happens naturally as we age, and you have a formula for wrinkles and looser skin. Hormones can affect the skin's physiology, with almost 30 percent of the skin's collagen depleted the first five years after menopause.

When I discovered that changing hormones were to blame for the acceleration of wrinkles and saggy skin, I ran to my doctor hoping for a huge dose of estrogen. What I discovered is that the FDA has not approved estrogen therapy to treat aging skin. There is no hard science to prove estrogen therapy can improve the appearance of your skin. I personally saw visible changes when I began hormone therapy. I know for a fact that hormone therapy alleviated my miserable symptoms; perhaps my *feeling* better had a positive effect on my complexion.

If you were a sun worshipper, a smoker or had bad eating habits, this can deplete more moisture, causing deeper wrinkles. If you used birth control pills or are currently on hormone therapy, you may be battling brown spots. Many women find new wrinkles cropping up, such as deep lines from smiling or frowning. Combine these frustrations with the fact that your skin's natural process of exfoliation called desquamation in which old cells slough off to make way for the new, and you have a dull looking complexion. As if that were not enough, you can thank gravity for all that sagging. Recently a menopausal friend asked, "If I hang upside down in gravity boots for an hour a day, will it stop the sagging?" Sadly, the answer is "no." Maybe a lifetime in space is the only answer to zero gravity.

HOW WILL YOU AGE?

We can't stop the aging process – even those of you running to the plastic surgeon cannot escape. I went on a beauty quest that would *embrace* my age, not disguise it. If you begin good beauty habits today, you can actually slow down the effects of aging.

Wouldn't it be nice to wave a magic wand and turn aging skin into youthful radiance? You cannot stop aging. Sorry, ladies, it bummed me out too. You can, however, manage aging. Embrace the experience by arming yourself with the magic of good beauty habits.

There are two types of aging--internal and external. Our genes cause internal aging. Internal aging begins in our 20's, but signs do not appear for decades. Dry skin, fine wrinkles, thin skin, and loss of underlying fat are examples of internal aging. Although we cannot stop internal aging, thankfully we can at least slow down external aging. External aging adds to our naturally occurring internal aging. The sun, gravity, facial expressions, sleeping positions, and smoking are all external factors that accelerate aging.

The 25 age-embracing tips below do not include dermabrasion, laser resurfacing, microdermabrasion, or chemical peels-- procedures that produce a new top layer of skin, removing brown spots and fine wrinkles. We can slow the aging process with good beauty habits. Applying these anti-aging tips can erase years off your face

How Will You Age Quiz | 25 Anti-Aging Tips
Check off the age-embracing guidelines you practice

✓	#	25 ANTI-AGING TIPS
	1	Wear sunscreen daily. The sun is your biggest enemy. Apply sunscreen of SPF 15 or greater 20 minutes prior to going outside.
	2	Cleanse and moisturize your skin twice daily.
	3	Use a retinol night cream.
	4	Be sure to moisturize the delicate skin around your eyes. Facial moisturizers or a moisturizing face cream will do the job.
	5	Remove makeup every night before going to bed.
	6	Moisturize and exfoliate your neck, hands and body skin.
	7	Enjoy weekly hydrating facial masks.
	8	Use anti-aging and antioxidant products for your skincare system.
	9	Massage your skin. It is good for blood circulation, relaxes muscles, and can relieve signs of tiredness.
	10	If you smoke, STOP.
	11	Take omega-3 supplements.
	12	Limit alcohol consumption.
	13	Wear sunglasses. Squinting from the sun will only accelerate the manifestation of those lines around your eyes.
	14	Avoid sun tanning. If you want a tanned look, use a facial bronzers or sunless tanners for a healthy summer glow.
	15	Avoid really hot showers and baths.
	16	Use detergent-free soaps for your face and body.
	17	Use 2% hydroquinone topical over-the-counter cream to lighten subtle skin discoloration.

18		Treat yourself to a professional facial, and discuss a skincare regime for your skin type.
19		Practice relaxation techniques. Second to sun damage, stress can age your skin.
20		Always wear a hat in the sun.
21		Sleep on a satin pillowcase to avoid facial creases, and get enough sleep.
22		Drink plenty of water.
23		Eat a healthy diet rich in antioxidants (citrus fruits, blueberries, strawberries, green tea, red vegetables, fresh salads). Avoid salt, sugar, caffeine and fatty foods. Eat fiber. Take your supplements. Eat fish 3-4 times per week.
24		Exercise most days of the week.
25		Maintain a healthy weight.

The Results

✓	#	HOW MANY TIPS DID YOU CHECK OFF?
	25	You go, girl. You will probably knock off 15 years from your age with these perfect beauty habits. Keep up the good work.
	20	Very impressive. Do people ask if your daughter is your sister? Kick it up a notch and join your sisters in the "25" group. Or stay where you are and your good habits will knock off 10 years.
	15	A good start. Add a few more tips, and join the ladies who ranked above you. Or continue the same strategy and notice 5 years knocked off your age.
	10	Nice try, but you won't see the results you may be looking for as the years pass. Try adding 5 tips monthly to your regime for the next 2-3 months.
	5	Oh, girlfriend…you either have great genes, or look like your grandmother. There is hope. Start adding some tips to your daily life, and fast. Depending on external factors in your life, it is never too late to begin practicing better grooming habits.
	0	What freedom to not worry about your skin. That could be a good thing. But one of these days, you'll wish you'd taken better care of your skin! Warning: Wake up and slap on some sunscreen and moisturizer.

◇◇

BEAUTY IS MORE THAN SKIN DEEP – BEAUTY RADIATES FROM A HAPPY SPIRIT AND HEALTHY BODY!

◇◇

SKINCARE SOLUTIONS THAT TURN BACK THE CLOCK

Many women visit their dermatologist or plastic surgeon to remedy new wrinkles and saggy skin. I have witnessed many friends go through uncomfortable injections for wrinkles, chemical peels, and full facelifts only to be disappointed with the results. Not only were many of these procedures expensive, they were painful and involved weeks or months of recovery time.

Daily moisturizing, weekly exfoliation, and wearing sunscreen can actually help turn back the clock of age, soften deep wrinkles and prevent brown spots. Weekly exfoliation can renew a dull complexion instantly. Moisturizing can soften wrinkles. If you want faster results, you can see a dermatologist—see the Getting Professional Help section on page 91. First, let's review non-surgical options available to maintain a healthy radiant skin.

NO MATTER YOUR AGE

Each age group has new skin concerns to address with an updated skin regime.

IN YOUR 30'S: Fine lines around the eyes. Frown and smiling lines begin to appear. Sleeping lines take longer to disappear. Spider veins may appear. You may begin to notice puffy eyes in the morning. Keep skin hydrated, and start using SPF 15+ daily.

IN YOUR 40'S: Facial expression lines become deeper. The bags under your eyes are more prominent; your skin becomes drier and more sensitive; your neck looks crêpe; your pores increase in size; increase or decrease in facial hair; age spots, spider veins, rosacea and saggy skin.

IN YOUR 50'S: Skin loses its elasticity faster. Wrinkles and deep folds may develop. The skin Becomes thinner and more fragile. You may develop "jowls" where the skin on the cheeks sags and hangs down either side of the chin. Sun damage is unforgiving now; brown spots increase, as well as deep lines in the cheeks and around the eyes and mouth. The eyelids may also have developed a crêpy appearance.

IN YOUR 60'S AND BEYOND: Dry, itchy skin. Age-spots, wrinkles and expression lines are etched into the face. Skin texture is not longer moist or supple. Skin is fragile and care must be taken to not tear it.

YOUR NEW SKINCARE REGIME

The skin is made up of two layers: The outer layer is called the "epidermis" and the inner layer is called the "dermis." The inner layer contains nerve endings, blood vessels, sweat glands and the collagen and elastin that support your skin. The epidermis produces melanin (pigment that is naturally present to varying degrees), and is constantly producing new skin cells to replace the ever-flaking dead skin cells. The skin is our body's protection from the environment – it regulates body temperature, stores water and fat, and prevents the entry of bacteria. Our skin is an important organ, and it is the one organ every can see. We all want beautiful healthy skin.

Even if you have already started to notice some wrinkles, you can soften them with a new skincare regime. Beauty tips that worked before your menopausal transition will need to be updated. Intensive moisturizing, using anti-aging products with retinoid and antioxidant ingredients, consumption of water, exercise and a healthy diet can bring back your youthful luster inside and out.

During menopause you may experience dry, itchy skin as well as loss of skin elasticity. Beautiful skin begins with a good, daily skincare regime. Turn back the clock and reclaim your youthful skin with the correct skincare regime.

MENOPAUSE MAKEOVER SKINCARE REGIME

SKIN TYPE

NORMAL	OILY	DRY	SENSITIVE	DEHYDRATED
CLEANSER				
Gentle cleansing gel or milk applied morning and night	Gentle cleansing gel or milk used for normal skin applied morning and night	Cleanser lotion or cream for dry skin. Must be gentle applied morning and night	Gentle milk or cream cleanser applied morning and night	Gentle milk or gel cleanser applied morning and night
TONER				
Alcohol-free toner applied morning and night	Alcohol-free toner applied morning and night	Gentle alcohol-free toner applied morning and night	Mild toner for sensitive skin applied morning and night	Hydrating toner applied morning and night

MENOPAUSE MAKEOVER SKINCARE REGIME

SKIN TYPE

NORMAL	OILY	DRY	SENSITIVE	DEHYDRATED
DAY CREAM				
Start using a daily moisturizer with SPF 15+ applied daily	Light water-based moisturizer with SPF 15+ applied daily	Rich oil-based moisturizer with SPF 15+ applied daily	Gentle daily moisturizer with SPF 15+ applied daily	Hydrating water-based moisturizer with SPF 15+ applied daily
NIGHT CREAM				
Light nourishing night cream applied nightly	Use same daily moisturizer without sunscreen applied nightly	Oil-based moisturizer for night repair applied nightly	Wear your day cream at night applied nightly	Deep-moisturizing night skincare cream to restore moisture loss applied nightly
EXFOLIATE				
Use an exfoliating scrub or glycolic at 2% applied 1-2 times weekly	Use an exfoliating scrub applied two to three times weekly	Fine scrub, mask, or glycolic at 2% applied once weekly	Use delicate exfoliate, if skin too sensitive do not exfoliate applied one to two times weekly	Exfoliating scrub applied once weekly
MASK				
Nourishing mask, alternate with deep cleansing mask applied 1-2 times weekly	Deep cleansing mask applied twice weekly	Oil-based mask applied one to two times weekly	Soothing mask applied once weekly	Nourishing mask applied once weekly

SKINCARE TIPS

- If you have combination skin, treat T-zone area with oily skin regime, and outside T-zone with either normal or dry regimes.
- If you skin is mature, treat using the dry skincare regime.

TELL YOURSELF "I AM HEALTHY AND BEAUTIFUL" FIVE TIMES TODAY.

KEEPING ALL OF YOU BEAUTIFUL DURING MENOPAUSE

As we age, many of us focus on beautifying our faces, because it is the one area we can't hide. During menopause, it's time to take special care of all of you—pamper your neck, body and hands too:

HANDS: Apply daily hand moisturizer and use SPF 15.
BODY: Use shower gel and moisturize entire body daily. Avoid harsh body scrubs.
NECK: Practice your face regime on your neck daily.

How you age, and how you experience menopause will be different for everyone. Some women age gracefully, while others look 10 years older than their age. Lifestyle (exercise, diet, stress levels, sleep habits, and sun protection), medical history, genes and how we take care of our skin will be reflected in our skin. Your skin is the largest organ you have—take care of it.

Beyond a new skincare routine, I discovered that accepting and loving myself was the greatest "non-surgical" solution for beauty. After a couple years of being depressed over my new wrinkles and sagging skin, I actually started seeing the beauty in my age. When I looked in the mirror, instead of focusing on looking older, I decided I had earned every wrinkle on my face, and was damn proud of it.

MAKEOVER TIPS	
	• Visit your dermatologist and check moles regularly.
	• Meditate. Managing stress is the first step to beauty. Stress is an instant skin destroyer.
	• If you have sensitive skin use fragrance free, and hypoallergenic products, exfoliating very little.

GETTING PROFESSIONAL HELP

Most of us are too busy to wait for over-the-counter results, and would prefer running to the dermatologist for a fast beauty fix. Before we move forward with magical solutions, I want to repeat: "Beauty radiates from a happy spirit and healthy body," not a plastic surgeon. That said, there are some relatively non-invasive procedures that can help erase some of the most common signs of aging. Even with my newfound pride for wrinkles, I too ran to my dermatologist for some beauty magic after watching my once-radiant skin sag, spot and drop. After years of hormone use, I had large brown spots on my face and tiny spider veins on my legs. I could live with my minor wrinkles and sagging but the spots and veins had to go!

THE MOST COMMON SKIN COMPLAINTS ATTRIBUTED TO AGING ARE:

Wrinkles	Spider veins/legs	Blotchy complexion
Saggy skin	Rosacea	Hair everywhere, or disappearing hair
Facial veins/red spots	Brown spots/sun damage	Droopy eyelids with crêping skin
	Dry skin	

Last year almost 16 million surgical and non-surgical cosmetic procedures were performed in the USA, per the American Society for Aesthetic Plastic Surgery. Non-surgical procedures make up over 90 percent of the total. The most popular non-surgical procedure is Botox, followed by soft tissue fillers, laser skin resurfacing, and microdermabrasion. Thirty- to fifty-four-year-olds get the majority of cosmetic treatments; this is the time in our lives when we are most self-conscious about aging.

If you decide to see a dermatologist to reverse the signs of aging, understanding your options will help you successfully choose the correct technique for your budget. Did you know there are many ways to "unwrinkle" a wrinkle? You can fill it, plump it, relax it, peel it, or resurface it.

With so many options, what is a menopausal gal to do?

1. Make an appointment with a board-certified dermatologist. Get references.
2. Discuss your concerns (wrinkles, brown spots, veins).
3. Listen carefully to the doctor's suggestions. Ask these questions:
   What results can I expect?
   Do you have "before" and "after" shots of the procedure?
   How many times has this doctor performed the procedure?
   Is your skin type correct for the suggested procedure?
   What is the recovery time?
   Are there side effects and risks?
   Let the doctor know if you have a history of scarring or herpes –
   both can affect the treatment outcome.
   How long do the results last – is there follow-up work?
   How and where is the procedure performed; how long will it take?
   What will it cost?

4. Be prepared for the procedure. Do you need to schedule recovery time (hiding time)? Can you afford it? Is the suggested procedure best for you?

5. If you need a second opinion, get one. It is *your* face!

CRASH COURSE IN NON-SURGICAL TREATMENTS

Non-surgical cosmetic treatments won't stop the aging process, but they will help hide the effects of aging. First, decide what you want to "fix" - wrinkles, brown spots, sun damage, acne scarring, loose skin, skin texture, large pores, discoloration, rosacea, broken capillaries, spider veins, facial flushing, or scars. Fortunately, science has given us many technology options to manage these skin complaints. Your next step is to choose the technique to treat your anti-aging condition that fits with your time frame and budget. Here are the most common nonsurgical options.

TREATMENT OPTIONS

Lasers

Ablative laser treatments damage the skin's surface so that it can then rebuild. Lasers are used to treat wrinkles, brown spots, sun damage, acne scarring, large pores, skin tightening, and smooth skin texture. Cost can range from $750.00 to $5,000.00 per session and there is recovery downtime. Non-ablative laser treatments do not damage the top layer of skin. These lasers are used to smooth wrinkles, tighten skin, zap brown spots, improve rosacea, eliminate broken capillaries, and remove pigmentation and scarring. Costs can range from $250.00 to $2,000.00 per session. Most dermatologists offer package deals.

What's the difference? Ablative has longer lasting effects, and you usually need just one treatment. But they are more expensive and the recovery takes longer. Non-ablative treatments, such as radio frequency and intense pulsed light, usually require four to six sessions and require little or no down time. Each session costs less, but you need more treatments to get the same results of the ablative treatments.

Chemical Peels

There are three categories of chemical peels: Light, medium, deep. Peels work by damaging the skin's surface to induce exfoliation through the application of various chemical agents. Light peels are used to smooth dull uneven skin, reduce the effects of sun damage, improve acne scars, soften fine wrinkles and remove brown spots. There is no downtime, but you may need multiple sessions. Medium peels are used to reduce large pores, soften acne scars, tighten skin, soften wrinkles, lessen brown discolorations, and repair sun damaged skin. Downtime is two to three days, and you may need multiple treatments. Deep peels are used for deeper wrinkles, wrinkling around the lips and chin area and sun damage. Downtime is one to two weeks with long-lasting results. Costs range from $150.00 to $300.00 for a light peel. Medium peels range from $1,500.00 to $2,500.00. Deep peels range from $2,500.00 to $3,000.00.

SOLUTIONS FOR BROWN SPOTS

Are you seeing spots? You are not alone, many women get brown spots during pregnancy, while taking birth control pills or during menopause due to the reaction of hormones or medications, and the biggest offender - the sun. If you have been exposed to the sun, are taking medications and/or going through hormone fluctuations, you have options to regain and keep your healthy glow:

1. Prevention, prevention, prevention: use sunscreen and wear a hat outside

2. Skin-lightening creams (Prescribed 4% hydroquinone creams. Over-the-counter 2% hydroquinone creams: Porcelana and Esoterica. These options take time to show results)

3. Use a tretinoin topical (acid form of vitamin A, the generic term for the medication Retin-A). Other brand names: Rejuva-A, Retisol-A and Renova

4. Laser therapy

5. Intense Pulsed Light (IPL)

6. Chemical peels

7. Microdermabrasion

8. Exfoliate using a glycolic acid

9. Eat antioxidant foods: yellow veggies, blueberries, cherries, blackberries and fresh fruits

10. Use antioxidant facial products

DERMABRASION

This ablative treatment uses a small rapidly spinning wheel with a roughened surface to remove the upper layers of skin. Dermabrasion is good for acne scars, wrinkles, brown spots and sun damage. It is long lasting, but you will need seven to 10 days of recovery time. Costs range from $200.00 up.

MICRO-DEMABRASION

This ablative treatment uses diamond chips to smooth away fine lines, uneven skin, age spots and acne scars. There is no downtime, but the results are temporary. Costs range from $150.00 and up.

DERMAL FILLERS

Many women choose dermal fillers for wrinkles around the eyes, frown lines, scars and lip enhancement. The dermatologist injects the area to be treated with a product that enhances soft tissue volume, adding extra fullness. This treatment usually lasts three to six months depending on the product used. Costs are typically $550.00 and up depending the location and amount used per session.

RELAXERS

One of the most popular treatments-- you probably know it as Botox--to soften wrinkles around the eyes and frown lines. Relaxers are injected under the skin and usually lasts three to six months. Costs range from $380.00 to $500.00 per session.

All of these non-surgical options offer immediate and visible results. Since cosmetic treatments are usually elective (not medically necessary), they are out-of-pocket expenses. These options may give you a head start on maintaining your youthful appearance. You will need to repeat treatments to maintain the same results over a longer period of time. Also, be aware that these treatments can carry risks. Speak to your doctor about potential side effects.

TAKING MORE DRASTIC ACTION: SURGICAL OPTIONS

If you want to erase years off your face, and can afford it, you may need to consider a surgical face-lift. These procedures are costly, and have a longer healing period and more risks. Ask yourself, "Is looking 10 years younger worth the risks of surgery? Can I maintain my skin with non-surgical options and practice good daily skin regime?"

ERASE YEARS OFF YOUR FACE – EXFOLIATE

Every 28 days your skin renews itself, leaving a fresh layer of baby skin cells. But as we get older, this shedding process – called "desquamation" – slows down, leaving us with fine lines, dry areas and an uneven skin texture. Makeup can really accentuate this dilemma.

Exfoliation stimulates new cell growth by removing the cells your body is no longer shedding. It helps your body with the desquamation process by stripping the dead epidermal cells off the outer surface of your skin, and exposing a fresher layer of living cells. It takes a few days for a noticeable amount of dead cells to accumulate. It is best to exfoliate once or twice a week. You do not want to irritate your skin or remove healthy living cells by exfoliating too much.

Exfoliation can benefit the skin on your face, as well as around your lips, neck, elbows, knees and feet. As I have gotten older, I have noticed the skin on my heels starting to crack – and the skin on my elbows seems thicker. Most of these dilemmas have improved as a result of exfoliating. For those of you who love to self-tan, exfoliation will be your best friend. It gives your skin a smooth texture, ensuring an even tan.

There are three different exfoliating methods:

* Manual: Manually scrub off the dead cells.
* Chemical: Dissolve with chemicals the glue-like substance that holds the dead cells together.
* Enzyme: Dissolve with enzymes the glue-like substance that holds the dead cells together.

They all work equally well. I was absolutely amazed at the results of administering such an inexpensive and simple process on my skin. Don't forget to exfoliate your elbows and feet; the benefits are immediate.

LOVING YOUR LOCKS

Why do women fuss with their hair and guys usually do not? Well, the answer is thousands of years old. In many cultures, a woman's locks represented status and sexual availability. Just as a man may strut his strength and money, a woman used her beauty—and her long, healthy hair—to attract a suitable partner. When we enter menopause and start noticing thinning hair, unwanted hair on our face, thinning eye lashes and graying hair, it is no surprise it causes anxiety.

WHERE DID MY HAIR GO?

Forty to 50 percent of women report some hair loss or thinning during menopause. Thinning hair and hair loss can lower self-esteem and cause embarrassment. The most common form of female hair loss is genetic, called *androgenic alopecia* (AGA), which is the same as male pattern baldness. Female hair loss during menopause can be cause for many different factors—genetics, age, fluctuating hormones and stress. Other, non-menopausal medical issues can cause hair loss, too. If you're concerned your thinning hair is due to a different condition, be sure to visit your doctor for a correct diagnosis.

COMMON REMEDIES FOR FEMALE HAIR LOSS

There are things you can do to help:

ROGAINE: FDA-approved, over-the-counter preparation of topical minoxidil (2 percent). This treatment helps to enlarge and lengthen your hair follicle, which extends the growth phase of your hair. This topical treatment does not cure hair loss, but can slow down the hair loss process.

SUPPLEMENT YOUR NATURAL HAIR: Wigs, hairpieces, or hair additions such as hair weaves.

HAIR TRANSPLANT SURGERY: Transplant surgery is an option, although it is expensive, can be painful, and takes up to two years to complete.

DRINK TEA: Some claim that consuming green tea helps, although this hasn't been proven.

SPECIAL SHAMPOO: Some women find that using shampoos containing hyaluronic acid can retard hair loss, but there is no scientific evidence that this works.

WHERE HAVE MY EYELASHES GONE?

What?! No more batting your eyelashes to the cute guy next to you? Just as we can start losing hair on our heads, your eyelashes can thin as well.

Good news is there are solutions. Depending on the severity, you may consider dying your lashes. Some mascaras claim to enhance eyelash appearance. Many women have false eyelashes fitted, but make sure they do not irritate your skin making eyelash loss worse. If you suspect your eyelashes many be thinning because of allergies, change your eye make-up and eye cleanser. Revitalash™ is a popular eyelash conditioner that yields thicker fuller looking eyelashes in just four weeks. If you are dealing with health issues discuss your thinning eyelashes with your healthcare provider. There is no need to lose your luscious lashes during menopause.

WHY DO I HAVE WHISKERS?

Over 40 million women in the United States alone have unwanted facial hair. Unwanted facial hair may appear as part of the normal aging process, as well as a result of fluctuating hormones as we go through menopause. Some women may only experience a few stray hairs on the chin, while others may grow visible hair on the upper lip. A small percentage of menopausal women who may develop a heavy, beard-like growth called hirsutism. Whether your growth is slight or extremely obvious, excessive facial hair can cause self-consciousness, and embarrassment.

There is nothing worse than looking in the mirror and finding a black hair growing out of your chin or a mole or worse – out of your forehead. What makes this experience so disturbing is that hair was probably growing there for the past week and everyone but you noticed it. During menopause there are a couple of causes for these unwanted facial visitors. Hormone fluctuations are one cause for increased facial hair. Women have both estrogens (female hormones) and androgens (male hormones, such as testosterone). As we age and enter the menopause transition, the levels of both hormones change, causing unwanted facial hair growth.

HOW DO YOU MANAGE OR TREAT UNWANTED FACIAL HAIR?

Women have been looking for ways to permanently remove hair for years. There are three different strategies to manage unwanted facial hair:

Temporary Removal	Medications	Permanent Removal
• Plucking • Bleaching • Chemical depilatories • Shaving • Waxing • Threading	• Vaniqua™ (not available in Canada)	• Laser and intense pulsed light (IPL) • Electrolysis • Hormone treatment • The birth control pill

Unwanted hair can be managed once you find a solution that works for you. Some women have great success with plucking a few stray hairs and bleaching the upper lip; others must resort to more aggressive and expensive methods to conquer unwanted hair.

BEAUTY SECRETS TO LOOK YOUR BEST

As our bodies change inside and out we need to adapt our beauty secrets. Practicing new beauty tricks can update your image. With a new hairstyle, updated make-up, and a brighter smile you can spice up your makeover so you look and feel like a new you. I felt ten years younger after I bleached my teeth, and my completion looked more radiant using a new light-reflecting foundation. After an updated hair cut and color adjustment I felt fashionable and sassy. Waterproof mascara can save the day if you are suffering from hot flashes!

~~~

FOCUS ON WHAT MAKES YOU BEAUTIFUL.

~~~

A NEW HAIRSTYLE CAN MAKE YOU LOOK AND FEEL YOUNGER

Whether you are losing your hair, or wishing it were not growing on your face, getting a new hairstyle can completely update your style. Many of us have had the same hairstyle and color for the past 10 to 20 years. What made you look hot 20 years ago will probably need revamping today. I have had the same hair color and cut most of my life. Menopause weight gain caused my face shape to become rounder, and the onset of rosacea changed my complexion tone. With warm-tones woven in my hair, and a new hairstyle I felt and looked years younger. For women dealing with hair loss, a shorter style offers more volume. For those with too much hair, a longer layered style will balance your face with your locks. Your hairstyle can completely transform your look.

HAIR COLOR

Don't fret about gray hair! If you are just getting a few gray strands, plucking is an easy and immediate solution. Or select a new hair color that is perfect for your complexion. A new hairstyle with a flattering color is a wonderful way to express your individuality, and look years younger! If you have a beautiful head of gray or silver, embrace it. Gray hair can be elegant.

How do you pick a hair color that is best for you? First, you must determine if your complexion is either "warm" or "cool" in tone. An easy way to find out is to look at the veins in your arms in natural light. If your veins look green you are warm, if they look blue you are cool.

Review this chart to confirm, and note the suggested hair colors for your category.

	COOL CATEGORY	WARM CATEGORY
EYES	Black-brown, dark-brown, dark blue, gray-blue, hazel with white, gray or blue flecks	Golden brown, hazel with gold or brown flecks, turquoise, green-blue
HAIR	Blue-black, ash brown, ash blonde, deep brown, platinum blonde	Red, strawberry blonde, gray-yellow, deep brown with gold or red highlights
SKIN	Very dark brown, true olive, medium with golden undertones, pale, bronze, medium pale	Pale with golden undertones, freckled, brown with pink or golden undertones, peachy or with peachy undertones, ruddy

Updating your hairstyle and color is a fun and easy way to boost your self-esteem. If you are feeling insecure about the menopause mid-section, a new hairstyle will bring the attention up to your face!

MENOPAUSE MAKE-UP SECRETS

A few makeup tips can enhance your appearance, and make you look and feel years younger. Makeup habits that worked for you in the past may need some updating to diminish the signs of aging. Generally speaking, it's better to go for a natural look. With more natural color tones and application, you'll look fresh and healthy—and younger! There are also many anti-aging makeup products available, such as SPF makeup and anti-aging foundations packed with antioxidants. Focus on your positive features, and let your natural beauty shine using new makeup tips.

Foundation

- Use moisturizer before applying foundation. If you have dry skin, apply a little face moisturizer to your makeup sponge, then apply foundation.

- Choose the correct color (ask an expert at the makeup counter for confirmation). Never buy foundation darker than your skin tone.

- Choose a foundation for your skin type. For oily skin, use an oil-free foundation; for dry skin, use a foundation rich in moisture.

- Purchase foundation with SPF 15+ unless you are wearing a moisturizer with SPF.

- Try an illuminating or light-reflecting foundation. It will brighten your skin, and make you look years younger. These products contain microscopic particles to reflect light.

- Use a sponge to apply foundation to a clean face and neck. Apply foundation in the center of your face and blend outwards, avoiding fine lines.

- Only apply foundation where needed. Often just applying foundation to the chin, cheeks and forehead will give you coverage for a fresh look.

- Blend foundation around the chin and neck areas.

- Remember: Less foundation is better than more; too much makeup can settle in your fine lines.

- Hot flash foundation advice: too much foundation is unforgiving during a hot flash. There are sweat-proof foundations and primers available, but the less foundation you wear the better. Carry facial blotting papers, a hand fan and touch-up foundation to freshen up after a hot flash attack.

- After you have applied your foundation, rub your palms together. Then press them onto your face. The warmth from your hands not only feels good, but also softens the foundation.

- Lightly mist your face with water to freshen up your makeup throughout the day.

Concealer

- Purchase a concealer with a yellow tone lighter than your natural skin tone.

- Moisturize your skin before applying concealer.

- Use your ring-fingertip to gently pat the concealer under the eyes and other areas that need coverage.

- Apply concealer from the inside of the nose, up to the lash line and on the dark areas under your eyes. Do not apply concealer on the eyelid.

- You can also use concealer on blemishes, scars, and brown spots.

- There are waterproof concealers for those suffering from hot flashes.

Powder

- Avoid powder if you can. It will accentuate facial hair and wrinkles.

- If you choose to wear powder, purchase a translucent powder with a matte finish.

- If you like the matte look powder offers, plus the benefit of setting your foundation use sparingly. If you suffer from hot flashes your powdering effort may need to be repeated after every hot flash. Hot flash sufferers should beware: the more make-up you wear, the more will sweat off during a hot flash. Less is better.

Lips

* Choose light and warm colors. Darker lipsticks accentuate problem areas and can make you look harsh.
* Line your lips with a lip pencil or lip liner before adding lipstick or lip gloss. Use a soft lip pencil with a wider tip so you can blend the lip's edges.
* Wear a lip balm with SPF 15+.
* Select natural-colored lip glosses.
* Avoid bright colors and frosted lipsticks.
* To make your lips appear fuller, you can add a touch of gloss to the inside of the bottom part of the lip.
* Use lip products with an emollient to keep lips soft. Also use balm to moisturize lips at night.
* If your lipstick bleeds during the day, apply powder to lips before putting your lipstick on.
* Use a lip brush when applying lipstick.

Eyes

* Choose lighter, warm, earthly tones. Purchase eye shadows that have 2-3 tones in the palette.
* Once you select a color tone, work with the 2-3 colors in that palette. Darkest color goes on your eyelid. Medium-color eye shadow goes in the eye socket, and the lightest color towards the outer corner of the eyebrow. Blend all the shades.
* Use eye shadows with a matte finish (frosty shadows will attract light and draw attention to those wrinkles you wish to disguise).
* Avoid bright colors and frosted shadows.
* Shadows are better than creams. Creams will settle in eye creases.
* Use an eye shadow brush to apply.
* Curl your eyelashes to open eyes. Use a lash curler just after your shower. Your lashes are easier to curl when they are warmed up after your shower.
* Finish your eyes with mascara, selecting a natural color. First coat, apply a volumizing formula starting from the base of your lashes. Then apply the second coat of lengthening mascara. Purchase waterproof mascara—there's no need for raccoon eyes even if you're having hot flashes!
* If you like to define your eyes, use eyeliner. Brown or charcoal may be better choices than black. Waterproof eyeliners are available if you are suffering from hot flashes.

* Always remove eye makeup before going to bed.
* If you have sensitive eyes, purchase hypoallergenic makeup
* Keep brushes clean.

Cheeks

* Use blush to contour your face.
* Avoid bright pinks; instead, use softer browns and peaches.
* Do not use too much blush. After applying blush to your brush, tap excess off brush before applying.
* Avoid blush with sparkles.
* To determine where to apply blush; bend over for 30 seconds; when you stand up, note where your natural color appears on your cheeks. Apply blush in this area, and then brush and blend outwards.

You don't have to be a makeup artist to find your natural beauty. If you need a second opinion, set up a makeup consultation appointment at your local department store. These professionals can offer tips, and confirm the best colors for you. With all the new anti-aging products flooding the market, a professional can give you samples to try before you make a purchase.

DRESSING THE NEW YOU

There are more than 40 million women over size 14, and by the year 2025 over 1.1 billion women will be going through menopause. Shopping for a new outfit can be frustrating when your body is changing as fast as your hormones and designers are focusing on younger smaller woman.

No matter what your size or shape, there are styles to flatter what you've got, and minimize what you don't. The first step to revamping your wardrobe is to identify your shape and note the styles that flatter your shape. Then clear all the unflattering clothes you have been wearing from your closet and go shopping! Bring a friend and a list of the clothes that flatter your body type.

MAKEOVER TIP:	Update your hairstyle and color before going shopping.

WHAT TO WEAR—AND WHAT NOT TO WEAR—FOR YOUR FIGURE

	Hourglass Classic curvy with large bust and hips, and a narrower waist	**Ruler** Chest, waist and hips are equal measurements, smaller bust	**Apple** Fuller in the middle
Tops	Fluted sleeves. Wrap tops. Fitted jackets. Blouses with defined waistlines. V-neck, scoop necklines. Tailored tops	Bold colors. Jackets with wide lapels and pockets that flare from waist. Strapless tops Vests. Ruffles	Tailored jackets with simple flare. Tops tighter under the bust line. Wide neck or wrap tops.
Bottoms	A-line skirts. Flare or boot-cut pants with flat front.	Boot-cut pants. Wide-legged pants. Wear shoes with heels	Wide-legged pants. With flat front
Dresses	Wrap dresses. Hem at knee or mid-calf, if you are tall	Shirt dresses with breast pockets. High-waisted dresses. Wear belt over or just below waistline	Styles that fall softly from bustline and have a flare just below the knee
Tips	Emphasis on natural curves. Choose narrow clothing lines	Create curves. Use scarves, belts, accessories	Draw attention towards neck with scarves, accessories and rounded collars
No-Nos	Tucks and gathers. Bulky fabrics. Too much detail around the bust. Spaghetti straps or halter tops. Too many accessories	Plunging necklines. Tapered pants. Boxy styles. Tight tops	Demin jackets. Pleated pants. Shiny fabrics around belly

WHAT TO WEAR—AND WHAT NOT TO WEAR—FOR YOUR FIGURE

	Petite	Pear	V-Shaped
	Shorter height with narrow hips and tiny shoulders	Upper body is smaller than your lower body. Hips larger than shoulders	Shoulders are 2" wider than hips. Fuller breasts, long legs.
Tops	Strapless tops. Focus on the waist or bust with ruffles, scarves and belts	Tailored tops. Jackets and tops hit narrow part of waistline or mid-thigh. Scoop neck, v-neck, rounded or square necklines. Puffy sleeves	Jackets that flare at hem. Shawl collars. Round or v-neck
Bottoms	Boot-cut pants with high pockets	Wraps and A-line skirts, hem at knee. Pants at waistline or just below. Boot-cut	Skirts or pants with flare. Wear belt lower than your waistline. A-line skirts. Boot-cut pants. Hipster jeans. Fitted tops
Dresses	Solid colors, hem at knee	Hem at knee. A-line dresses. Flare hem	Hem at knee. A-line dresses
Tips	Dress mono-chromatically	Wear darker colors on bottom. Soft patterns on top	Show off legs. Wear sexy shoes. Wear bright colors and thicker fabrics on bottom. No scarves or bulky accessories
No-Nos	Shoulder pads. Long skirts. Ankle straps on shoes. Big prints	Tight clothes. Busy patterns on bottom. Pant side pockets	No baggy pants. No skinny jeans

MAKEOVER TIPS:

- Choose colors that flatter your skin tone.
- Dark colors minimize.
- Patterns and bright colors bring attention.
- Avoid narrow-ankle pants.
- Avoid high-waisted outfits – they'll make you look bigger in the middle or even pregnant.
- Purchase an outfit that flatters your body, not necessarily one that fits in with the latest hot trend.

No matter what your body shape, during menopause your waistline may get larger. For the past year I have been hiding my disappearing waistline with baggy clothes. With body fat shifting to the belly, it's time for a shopping spree!

12 STYLING TIPS

1. Wear clothes that fit; baggy clothes will only make you look bigger.

2. Measure yourself so you know what size to buy.

3. Monochromatic outfits are slimming. Dressing in one color is always flattering and classy.

4. Add color and accent with accessories, scarves, blazers or cardigans. Necklaces should be worn long. Scarves should be long and tied loosely.

5. Any stripes should be vertical.

6. If you wear a belt, it should be light and feminine. A bulky heavy belt can "shorten" you.

7. Wear a heel on your shoe. Feeling and looking taller is always a winner.

8. Choose darker colors for your basics. Navy, charcoal, gray and black are slimming.

9. Undergarment foundations are my newest discovery this year! I purchased an all-in-one shaper so I was firmer and my soft lumpy spots didn't ruin a nice line in an outfit.

10. Know your best feature. If it is your legs, wear knee-length dresses. If it is your bust, enjoy a plunging neckline. Whatever your special asset, this is the time to flaunt it.

11. Carry an oversized handbag. Proportion can fool the eye. Square-shaped bags look good on rounder figures, and a purse with a strap should not land in your "problem" areas.

12. Once you update your wardrobe, add a few sexy shoes, a fun handbag and accessories for day and nighttime.

UNDERGARMENTS

Spoil yourself with romantic sleepwear and undergarments. Not for "him" but for you. When I was feeling fat, frumpy and hormonal, I went out and purchased some sexy underwear and PJ's. When I wore the sexy underwear I felt like I had a little secret that no one knew about but me. I smiled all day wearing my pretty panties and felt confident that I possessed the experience and knowledge that only comes with age. And at night, I felt sassy slipping into a feminine outfit. Try it!

THE CORRECT FITTING BRA CAN MAKE YOU LOOK PERKY – AND LOOK 10 POUNDS LIGHTER IN LESS THAN FIVE MINUTES.

HOW TO PROPERLY FIT A BRA

Almost 80 percent of all women are wearing the wrong size bra. A bad fitting bra can make you look frumpy, and lumpy. One of the smallest areas of our midsection is just under our boobs. Don't hide a thinner area with droopy boobs--lift those "sisters" and show off that sexy area. Many of us have continued to wear the same size bra for decades, despite our changing bodies. Many women have never been properly measured and fitted for the correct size bra. With aging your body shape may change, as well as your bra size. When we shop for bras we hunt for styles we like, but the fit is just as important.

Size Matters

It is easy to properly fit a bra. First, determine your chest size or band size (32, 34, 36, 38, etc.). Second, determine cup size (A, B, C, D, CC, DD, etc.).

Step One: Band Size

Wear your best-fitting bra, and measure directly under the breast. Exhale when measuring. Round up to a whole number. If the number is even, add four inches. If the number is odd, add five inches. This is the band size.

Step Two: Cup Size

Stand straight. Arms are your sides. Loosely measure at the fullest part of your breast while wearing a nonpadded bra. Do not wear a sports bra during measuring. Round up numbers to a whole number.

Step Three: Calculate Bra Size

Subtract the Step One band measurement from the Step Two cup measurement. If there is a half-inch measurement, increase the cup one size up.

(Cup sizes: AA = no difference, A = 1", B = 2", C = 3", D = 4", DD = 5", F = 6", G = 7", H = 8")

Once you've taken your measurements, go to the lingerie department of your favorite store and try on bras with your new calculations. Don't be afraid to ask for help from the lingerie salesperson.

MANICURES AND PEDICURES – LIFE'S LITTLE LUXURY

As the years pass, schedules fill up, and responsibilities preclude pampering time, we often forget to make time for manicures and pedicures. During your *Menopause Makeover,* schedule a manicure and pedicure weekly or semi-monthly. It is a wonderful way to make time for yourself. Take care of your hands and feet during menopause.

This chapter is dedicated to rediscovering your beauty, inside and out. Most of us have been practicing beauty tips from our teen years that no longer work during menopause. Cleansing habits, makeup application, purchasing properly fitted bras, wearing flattering styles, and personal grooming must all be updated when we go through "the change." We must change. In order to regain control of your beauty, you must embrace these changes as much as we did during our teen years.

You will increase your confidence and self-esteem with a new hip pair of glasses or sexy jeans, or a new flattering hairstyle. Menopause and aging do not have to signal the end of feeling beautiful. Instead, you can begin to find a new kind of beauty. Let your spirit shine-that is the greatest beauty tip of all. Don't let magazine advertisements, commercials and the media define beauty. We are all beautiful.

MAKEOVER TIPS	
	• Practice good posture, stand proud.
	• Manage unwanted hair.
	• Wear sunblock with SPF 15+.
	• Get your beauty rest.
	• Exfoliate weekly.
	• Cleanse and moisturize daily.
	• Use anti-aging products with retinoid and antioxidant ingredients.

MAKEOVER TIPS

* Update your makeup.
* Get a new hairstyle and color.
* Throw out old clothes, and replace with new flattering styles.
* Purchase new bras that fit properly.
* Don't forget to pamper your hands, feet, neck and body.

MAKEOVER TAKE ACTION LIST

* Update your skincare regime.
* Schedule a facial, and discuss skincare with the technician.
* Collect magazine clippings of hairstyles you like that would be good for your face shape.
* Make an appointment with your hairstylist.
* Schedule an appointment at your local department store beauty counter to discuss makeup tips and update your makeup.
* Select a teeth-whitening option.
* Buy a new properly fitted bra and cool pair of jeans.
* Make sure your closet has new basics and that old styles get tossed.
* Schedule a manicure and pedicure.
* Set beauty goals.

IN YOUR ESSENTIAL PLANNER

* Track beauty goals weekly in Your Weekly Progress report.
* Enter all appointments—spa, makeup artist, hairstylist—in Your Month-at-a-Glance planner to keep track of your makeover.
* Record your beauty connections in Your Menopause Makeover Contacts.

| Chapter 6 | Step Five: Am I Losing My Mind? Getting Off the Emotional Roller Coaster |

We've all heard the expression "mind over matter." Well, going through menopause will put you to the ultimate test. With so much happening to your body and your brain, some pretty big emotions get stirred up. These changes can make you irritable, cranky and sad – and feeling out of control over these uninvited changes. As if dealing with emotions weren't enough, my memory started to act a bit funny: some memories came flooding back and some just seemed to disappear completely.

This chapter addresses the emotional side of menopause—the symptoms and changing brain chemistry that can affect your daily life. It is often these changes that can make going through menopause so challenging. Going through menopause, whether you are perimenopausal or postmenopausal, can push some big emotional buttons. Ever-changing hormones can trigger moodiness that can open the door for previously hurt feelings to surface. Other feelings pop up from midlife and lifestyle changes. Throw in feelings fueled by confusing social expectations and our personal commitments, and watch out! Each section in this chapter will explain emotional challenges and offer you solutions to start feeling sane again. You'll come away with a better understanding of why you've been asking, "Have I lost my mind?"

YOUR IDENTITY

From childhood to young womanhood, each of us forms a unique identity. Women often choose between two common identifiers: marriage and motherhood, and/or a professional career. We have been fortunate during past 50 years to be able to have these choices. Now we have the choice to have children early or later in life, and can seek financial independence. When our biological clock ticks from the reproductive years into the freedom phase of menopause, we can choose to be stressed out because the baby-making chapter has ended, or we can celebrate our newly attained independence.

Menstrual cycles and childbearing have physical transitions just as menopause does, mostly driven by hormones. It is true that nine months of uncomfortable pregnancy symptoms are shorter than five to seven perimenopausal years, but the freedom from PMS, periods, birth control and worrying about everyone else can bring relief. The journey from perimenopause to postmenopause can challenge your self-image, self-esteem, and body image. This transition is a wonderful time to re-think your identity.

1. How do I define success (motherhood, career, finances, social status, relationships, charity)?

2. What dreams have I placed on the back burner, which can be reignited?

3. What makes me happy?

4. How do I feel about age? What is my greatest fear about growing older (wrinkles, weight gain, not being sexy, health concerns)?

5. How would I rate my self-esteem (1 to 10, with 10 being self-confident and happy)?

6. How can I improve my self-esteem?

7. How do I rate my body image (1 to 10, with 10 being smoking hot)?

8. How can I improve my body image?

9. How do I view myself? How do others view me?

10. If I could change one thing about my identity, what would it be?

YOUR MOTHER'S MENOPAUSE

Many years ago, our mothers had a very different menopausal transition. Most women did not discuss their troublesome symptoms. They suffered silently, and hoped "the change" would end sooner than later. When I asked a friend's mother about her menopause, she said, "Oh, it was no big deal." Then her daughter quickly reminded her about her hysterectomy, and the stressful period she had experienced going through menopause. Her mother had completely blocked out her menopausal experience. Many daughters duplicate their mother's physical journey, so understanding your mother's experience – both physically and emotionally – may help you gauge your own.

Women are overwhelmed with busy schedules in our fast-paced world. Throw menopause into the mix, and it can result in an extremely stressful time. Fortunately, a growing number of doctors and scientists in the United States today are women, and menopause research is on the rise. Menopause is finally "out of the closet."

If you can discuss menopause with your mother, it may assist during your experience. It may also give your mom a place to express buried feelings about her menopause transition.

QUESTIONS FOR MOM

1. What were your worst symptoms going through menopause?
2. Were you emotional?
3. Did you experience weight gain?
4. Did you have any medical conditions pop up during "the change?" High blood pressure? Bone density changes? Cancer?
5. How did you feel going through menopause?
6. Do you have any advice for me?

SOCIAL EXPECTATIONS

One of the biggest complaints among menopausal women is the frustration they feel from society's expectations. In the United States, as well as many European countries, women are valued for their youth and beauty. In the past, a woman's feminine beauty was considered to be *over* after menopause. No wonder our mothers did not discuss going through "the change!" Yet in other cultures, women are celebrated after they pass through menopause. Women are celebrated during this natural stage of life and are often welcomed into the "man's world" with open arms. In Asia, women are more respected after menopause, and can achieve a higher status in society. Age is a badge of honor, not a sign of worthlessness. Sadly, in other cultures, including our Western culture, the general attitude is that menopause is a loss of beauty and youth – and that equals a loss of sexiness and value.

Yet, there is hope! And it begins with us. A few brave advertisers, Dove™ being one of them, celebrate woman's physical passage through the different stages in her life. An estimated 6,000 US women reach menopause every day (over 2 million per year). We can choose to be embarrassed by the experience, or we can embrace the transition. We must let society know that we positively acknowledge this stage in our lives. This is the only way social beliefs, expectations and stereotypes will change – our voices must be heard. We, the baby boomers, have a loud voice. Let's use it! Then society will look at menopause as our celebration of entering into a new, liberating stage of life.

Many of us fear that men will no longer find us attractive. Men will continue to mirror our fear of aging, unless we start seeing beauty in ourselves.

HOW TO FIND YOUR MENOPAUSE SWAGGER

- Read biographies of great women who found success over the age of 40.

  I'm Not Slowing Down, by Ann Richards, former governor of Texas

  Cloris: My Autobiography, by Cloris Leachman, Oscar and nine-time Emmy Award winner

  Growing Up Again: Life, Loves, and Oh Yeah, Diabetes, by actress and activist Mary Tyler Moore

  Audition, by network diva Barbara Walters

  Age is Just a Number: Achieve Your Dreams At Any Stage In Your Life, by Olympic gold medalist Dara Torres

  I Feel Bad About My Neck, by writer Nora Ephron

- Make a list of your life accomplishments (graduating high school, college, marriage, children, career successes, winning a contest, travels).

- Make a list of five things you've always wanted to do (spend a week in bungalow in Tahiti, read English novelist Jane Austin's series of novel, pamper yourself at a spa retreat, learn to fly or sail, write poetry, skydive). Set a goal to do or start one a month or all five over the next year.

- Every morning stand in front of the mirror naked and say, "I am beautiful and sexy." So some things are droopy and lumpy these days – don't let your self esteem droop! Focus on your perfect self hiding under your fat suit. A firm self-esteem is stronger than a firm tush.

- Every day go out into the world knowing you are beautiful and sexy. How you feel about yourself says more to the world than your appearance.

- Find areas in your life that define you not driven by your looks—what are you especially proud of? What are you especially good at? Turn of the disparaging voice in your head and write down 10 things you've accomplished that make you feel great about yourself.

- Make a list of how you can make the world a better place. Maybe you could join a volunteer organization, or vow to drop groceries off for the elderly woman next door. Pick one thing from your list and go do it!

- If you had one month to live, what would you do? I doubt, it would be Botox or a tummy tuck!

- Don't let magazine ads influence your sense of self. Every time you start comparing yourself to a magazine ad, remember that the model was likely photoshopped beyond recognition!

- Treat yourself like royalty and you will feel royal. Pamper, pamper, pamper yourself. Get a pedicure, buy a new pair of shoes, or take a long soak in the tub.

- Don't forget to smile.

WHAT, ME, CRANKY AND MOODY?

Feeling cranky, irritable, impatient, and moody is common during menopause. The out-of-control and uninvited emotional outbursts are hard to live with. Some women experience higher levels of anxiety during menopause that can lead to panic attacks, dizziness, and heart palpitations. These attacks can be scary to the one suffering from them, as well as to loved ones witnessing these effects. Often we can thank fluctuating hormones for our wacky emotions. Throw in hot flashes, and vaginal dryness – no wonder you are cranky and moody!

HORMONES GONE HAYWIRE

Check all that apply to you.
When your hormones go haywire you feel:

- ☐ Cranky, irritable, moody
- ☐ Sad
- ☐ Impatient
- ☐ Unmotivated
- ☐ Fatigued

- ☐ Anxious
- ☐ Stressed
- ☐ Anxious
- ☐ Aggressive
- ☐ Like you have difficulty concentrating

WHEN YOU FEEL CRANKY, LIST THE THINGS YOU ARE THANKFUL FOR.

WHY THE ROLLER COASTER?

This menopause emotional roller coaster can happen for a variety of different reasons. Knowing the cause can help you find the solution. Speak to your practitioner if you think hormones are to blame and consider seeing a therapist if lifestyle changes have you feeling stressed. Among the factors that may be contributing to your menopausal moodiness:

* You may be suffering from hormone fluctuations. If you suffered from bad PMS due to menstrual hormones, menopause may feel like full-time PMS.

* You recently had a hysterectomy, causing your hormones to change drastically.

* You are not getting enough sleep because you're suffering from night sweats.

* You are experiencing stressful lifestyle changes, such as career change, an empty nest, or caring for aging parents.

* You have money/retirement fears.

* Your life is stressing you out. Career stress or relationship issues can make you moody or anxious.

* Loss of libido.

* You are upset at growing older. Your view of aging and menopause if negative or you feel grief at no longer being able to have children.

* Your medical health deteriorating.

* You have a history of clinical depression; the hormonal fluctuations of menopause can trigger depressed feelings.

HOW TO COPE

Discuss hormone therapy with your doctor, and consider the following strategies:

* Seek support from friends and family

* Find quiet time for yourself

* Meditate

* Take a yoga class

* Exercise

* Eat healthfully (higher protein, low-glycemic diet)

* Avoid alcohol or sedatives

* Discover new ways to creatively express yourself

* Don't smoke

* Make sure you get a good night's rest

* Pamper yourself

HORMONES AND THE BRAIN

The female brain goes through many changes over the course of a lifetime, largely thanks to changing levels of hormones like estrogen. In her book, *The Female Brain*, Dr. Louann Brizendine explains how the female brain changes from birth to puberty to motherhood to menopause due to changing hormones.

From birth, a girl's brain receives enormous amounts of estrogen. Dr. Brizedine says, "This high quantity of estrogen also stimulates the brain circuits that are rapidly being built…enhancing circuits and centers for observation, communication, gut feelings and caring." From the time we're little girls, estrogen is already helping us become fantastic communicators and empathizers.

Hormones play a significant role during puberty, too. As Dr. Brizendien explains how fluctuating hormones affect the turbulent teen years: "The rising tide of estrogen and progesterone starts to fuel many circuits…. assuring that … female-specific brain circuits will become even more sensitive to emotional nuance, such as approval and disapproval, acceptance and rejection. These changing circuits drive the way [a girl] thinks, feels, and acts [so] a girl's primary purpose is to become sexually desirable and attractive."

When a woman is pregnant there are huge increases in progesterone and estrogen. Her brain begins to focus on nesting and her brain is calmed by progesterone. As Dr. Brizenine says, "The mommy brain is switched on right at birth by a cascade of oxytocin." Oxytocin is the maternal bonding hormone, friend of dopamine that gives a woman those nurturing feelings. The mommy brain is committed to caretaking, putting the needs of her family over her own. Child rearing continues to be fueled by oxytocin as well as cycling estrogen, progesterone and testosterone.

Then during menopause our brains change again, as Brizendine explains, "The mommy brain unplugs. Menopause means the end of the hormones that have boosted communication circuits, emotion circuits, the drive to tend and care, and the urge to avoid conflict at all costs." During perimenopause, estrogen begins to decline, and so does oxytocin, the hormone responsible for connecting and caretaking. Menopause marks the time of low estrogen and no progesterone, where the brain circuits that were fueled by estrogen, progesterone and oxytocin are altered.

During menopause, a woman begins to focus on her health. During postmenopause there is more calmness because estrogen, testosterone and oxytocin are low and steady. A woman is less emotional and becomes more interested in what *she* wants to do and less on taking care of others. Most women experience a shift from caretaking to personal growth from perimenopause through post menopause.

After reading Dr. Brizendine's research, it all made sense. I wasn't losing my mind; my hormones were simply changing. Knowing that our mind chemistry changes, affecting our behavior and moods, soothed my fears. I felt validated knowing there was a scientific reason for the way I felt.

My brain rewired from mommy brain to independent brain, no longer driven by care taking. Of course, I still enjoy taking care of my loved ones, but it is different now. It is a choice, not an urge. What freedom! This new "menopause brain" offers us the opportunity to contribute not only to our families, but also to our communities. It can make you really feel like Wonder Woman™ – you can change the world with your new menopause brain. I decided to write this book with my new menopause brain! Menopause is your time to focus on *you*.

DEPRESSION

Women who have a history of depression may also suffer from depression during menopause. Some may experience depression for the first time during the menopause transition. Depression can make going through menopausal physical and emotional changes more difficult.

Clinical depression is defined as being intensely sad or feeling severe desperation that affects your daily life for more than two weeks. Clinical depression can silently rob your life of joy, happiness and healthy relationships. If you have a history of depression, have suffered from severe PMS or postpartum depression, or have a strong family history of depression, you may be at higher risk for clinical depression. Depression is a disease caused by very real biological conditions, including declining levels of estrogen and progesterone disturbing the levels of serotonin, medical conditions (heart disease, thyroid, sleep disorders or a head injury), and some prescription drugs.

In addition to physical reasons, depression has psychological causes as well. A significant loss (a divorce, death, new empty nest, or feeling a loss of youth) can trigger depression. Situational changes that may cause depression include changes in relationships, personal losses or crises, or overwhelming situations and life changes, all of which are common to menopause.

SYMPTOMS OF DEPRESSION

* Sadness
* Hopelessness
* Feeling desperate
* Tiredness
* Irritability

* Feeling worthless
* Feeling guilty
* Overly stressed about weight changes
* Loss of libido
* Changes in appetite

* Activities that used to make you happy no longer do
* Difficulty concentrating
* Sleeplessness
* Thoughts of hurting yourself

TREATMENTS FOR DEPRESSION

1. Pay attention to your moods; keep notes on how you feel in The Menopause Makeover journal.

2. Antidepressants can help depression. There are many different classes of antidepressants; most work by increasing levels of key neurotransmitters, such as serotonin, in the brain. Discuss this option, as well as other types of antidepressants, with your practitioner.

3. For some women, hormone therapy has a beneficial effect when added to other antidepressant treatment.

4. Psychotherapy can help resolve many issues contributing to your depression.

5. Exercise can make you feel better. Your body creates feel-good endorphins during aerobic activity that can help improve your mood.

6. Eat healthfully.

7. Avoid excessive alcohol and caffeine.
8. Pamper yourself (massage, facial, manicure, a trip out of town)
9. Get enough sleep.
10. Join a support group, and surround yourself with friends and support.

Often women suffering from depression don't even know it. If someone who loves you suggests you get help for depression, listen!

Depression can leave you feeling lethargic and unable to properly care for yourself. If menopause is combined with clinical depression, seek help with managing your depression and other menopause symptoms. Do not go through depression alone.

MEMORY LOSS

Have you ever been out doing chores when you receive a call from a friend who has been waiting an hour for your arrival, and you completely forgot? Or do you repeat yourself a few times, because you forgot you said it earlier, only to have it pointed out by your listener?

Sometimes short-term memory loss can occur when hormones fluctuate. Declining estrogen levels may affect the levels of the neurotransmitters dopamine and serotonin. A drop in these levels can lead to moodiness, fuzzy thinking, and short-term memory loss. Age, stress, medications and overall health can also contribute to short-term memory loss. Also, if you are exhausted after suffering from night sweats, and not getting enough sleep, it is no surprise if you become forgetful.

You are not crazy – ask for the support of your loved ones to nurture you through your forgetful moments. Get organized with planners, calendars and PDAs. Treating night sweats and hot flashes with low-dose hormone therapy may also help you feel sharper. Keep your mind active and enjoy a healthy lifestyle. Get enough sleep; a rested mind can absorb more information.

STRESS

We all experience stress. Daily stress triggers can include: Relationships, children, family, finances, work deadlines, traffic, busy schedules, and constantly ringing cell phones. Mix in menopause symptoms…and stress triggers can skyrocket. Hot flashes, aging, weight gain, midlife changes, empty nest, sleepless nights, and a low libido can all crank up the stress meter. Just when you need to be at your best to manage all this stress, your fluctuating hormone levels may affect the mood centers in your brain, causing you to melt down. Chronic stress can wreak havoc on your overall health and happiness.

WHEN YOU ARE STRESSED OUT

* It is difficult to lose weight
* You may experience migraines, irritable bowel syndrome, acid reflux, and back and joint pain
* You feel gloomy and tearful
* You have a hard time concentrating
* You are constantly irritable and cranky
* You feel hopeless
* Damage can be caused to your immune system, making you are susceptible to infections and viruses
* You have a harder time going through menopause

HOW TO COPE WITH STRESS

* Identify stress triggers, and resolve relationship issues.
* Try stress-relieving activities, such as yoga, meditation, or tai chi.
* Regular exercise releases endorphins, making you feel better.
* Schedule fun activities.
* Make time for your friends; support is important.
* Eat healthfully – avoid a diet heavy in carbohydrates.
* Pamper yourself a little bit—take a hot bath, or treat yourself to a manicure or massage.
* Get in touch with your spirituality (see chapter 8).
* Get plenty of rest.
* Slow down and take time in the day for yourself.
* Find a relaxing new hobby.
* Start reading more, and watch a little less television.
* Free up your schedule – start saying no to others, and yes to you.
* Make a point of laughing every day.
* Don't always answer your cell phone.
* Make fun plans for the weekend.
* And if you have a partner, a little affection and intimacy goes a long way – make sure *you* are satisfied.

For many of us, the menopause journey can be stressful. It's especially critical that you manage stress during menopause, so that you can take care of yourself. Once you handle stress triggers, managing menopause symptoms is possible.

Whether they are suffering from midlife issues, lifestyle changes, hormone fluctuations, social pressures or personal expectations, it is no surprise that women going through menopause are emotional! Make time daily to pamper yourself, and get rest. You are going through a major shift in your life. Everything you know is being altered, emotionally and physically.

If you cannot manage the emotions and stress in your life on your own, seek professional help. A therapist can help with many issues in your life, relationships, or past that may need to be addressed. Your practitioner can discuss the possibility of hormone therapy or the use of antidepressants. Some people find that the herb St. John's Wort can help counteract depression and stress, but if you take St. John's Wort, be sure to inform your doctor. This herb is often not compatible with other medications, and drug interactions can be dangerous.

CALL IN THE TROOPS

One of the greatest contributions you can make to help maintain your emotional health is to seek support from loved ones, friends or a psychotherapist. Add the names and contact informa-tion of your support team in the ultimate planner in Chapter 13.

Discuss treatment options with your doctor if you are suffering from depression, moodiness, emotional outbursts, forgetfulness and fuzzy thinking. Inform your healthcare provider of any genetic dispositions, health issues, and lifestyle or relationship changes.

MAKEOVER TIPS:

- Let your friends and loved ones know you are struggling with uncontrollable crankiness, moodiness and fuzzy thinking; ask for their support.
- When you start feeling a surge of out-of-control emotions building up – stop, breathe, count to ten. Take a "time out" for yourself.
- If you suspect these crazy emotions are hormonal, discuss hormone therapy and/ or antidepressants with your doctor.
- If your emotions are related to relationship or lifestyle concerns, schedule an appointment with a psychotherapist.

MAKEOVER TAKE ACTION LIST

- Spend time reviewing your answers to the Identity Questionnaire on page 110.

- Speak to your mother about her menopause experience. See suggested questions on page 112.

- Are you suffering from menopausal crabbiness, moodiness, depression or short-term memory loss? ___ Yes ___ No If yes, what solutions work for you? Refer to page 115 (how to cope with the crazy menopausal emotional roller-coaster).

- What can you do to cope with your stress? Refer to page 119.

- Identify and enter goals, pages 191 and 192.

- If you already have a busy schedule, start cutting back on your responsibilities. Make time for you.

IN YOUR ESSENTIAL PLANNER

- Schedule any take-action tasks on Your Month-at-a-Glance planner.

- If you are suffering from any abnormal emotions, depression or short-term memory loss, schedule an appointment with you doctor or physiotherapist.

- Make a list of friends you can call for support, record their contact information on page 209.

- In your 12-Week Plan, schedule quiet time.

- In your 12-Week Plan, schedule pampering time for yourself.

- Make note of any emotional outbursts in your 12-Week Plan.

- If you are suffering from depression, memory loss or stress document in your Medical Forms

- Journal your feelings daily

- List your support team and doctor contacts in Your Menopause Makeover Contacts

Chapter 7	Step Six: Why Are They All Running Away? Strengthen Your Relationships and Get that Sizzle Back into Your Sex Life

He stood frozen like a deer caught in the headlights of a car. His eyes bugged out and the hair on the back of his neck was standing at full attention. His shoulders hunched up around his ears. He was in full retreat mode. White as a ghost and trembling with fear, he worried that one step in the wrong direction could result in his own demise, or end his marriage. How did he get here? What happened? How could he escape?

Welcome to my husband's world. While my world was consumed with daily emotional avalanches and dreadful menopause symptoms, his world was filled with confusion. Ravaged by hot flashes, weight gain, cranky moods, lack of sleep, tender breasts, disappearing self-esteem and a dry vagina, I had lost my sense of compassion and understanding. I had become an erupting volcano of anger. After a few months, I wondered, "Why is everyone running away from me?"

For most women, loved ones are one of our greatest sources of satisfaction. The majority of our adult lives have been spent caring for others, and we tend to put ourselves second to those we love. You have probably given a large part of your life to your family. During menopause, your most beloved relationships could be tested.

Once you reach menopause, irritability may increase because the ratio of estrogen to testosterone starts shifting.

Fluctuating hormones can cause some serious crankiness. And keeping the peace no longer seems like the priority it was during your childbearing years. As our hormones change, we change emotionally too.

So, what's a menopausal soul to do? This chapter will present easy-to-understand explanations about how our changing hormones can affect our relationships, and offer some possible solutions. It also includes helpful hints for your guy and suggestions for what to say when you're in a rough spot. The Menopause Makeover can only be successful when your partner, family and friends understand what you are experiencing, so you can receive support.

NOTE

Acknowledging that relationships exist between women and men, and between women and women, this chapter has something for everyone. Because a female partner can have the advantage of relating to her menopausal lover differently than a man can, some of the information in this chapter is directed toward the male in the female/male relationship. Relationships with other loved ones, friends and co-workers, are also addressed here here.

RELATIONSHIPS AND SEXUAL HEALTH

"Honey, you are never *in the mood* anymore. It's been awhile, I really need to *get some*," he says staring at the ceiling in the dark.

She says, "It's always about *you*. What about *me*? I have been feeling like crap lately. I am exhausted; these night sweats keep me up all night. All I do is household chores, deal with your stuff, and work. Frankly, why is it always about you?"

He says, "Well, for the past 12 years, you never complained. I thought you liked to make love to me?"

She says, "Even if I was up for sex, my vagina is so dry it hurts every time we do it. Do you wonder why I am not in the mood? I would rather go shoe shopping than make love to you."

She rolls over, pulling up the covers. He rolls over. Facing away from each other, she stares into the darkness, angry and misunderstood. He kicks the sheets off his feet, frustrated and disappointed.

Some studies claim that guys between the ages of 20 and 32 think about sex every 52 seconds, and women think about sex once a day. As we enter perimenopause, the female sex drive can decline significantly, continuing through postmenopause. Over 50 percent of menopausal women may experience a lower sex-drive. As we age, the sexual desire gap between men and women may widen. For some women sexual desire can increase, but this is not as common. If you want to nurture a healthy relationship, you will have to address the declining libido issue.

Hormones can affect relationships physically and emotionally during menopause. Usually the partner in your life will notice your lack of libido before noticing that you are completely wretched from hot flashes.

When I asked a group of menopausal women between the ages of 41 and 54 if they still felt sexy during menopause, over half of them said no. I think the other half lied. The majority of women attributed their fading interest in wanting to "make whoopee" to:

- Feeling unattractive from weight gain.
- Declining libido.
- Vaginal dryness.
- Lack of sleep from night sweats and hot flashes.
- Moodiness.
- Not being happy.

- Feeling old, fear of aging.
- Being depressed.
- Being fatigued.
- Feeling isolated.
- Feeling a sense of loss at not being able to have children anymore.

How could anyone feel romantic with these all-consuming negative feelings combined with overwhelming menopause symptoms? Most of these mood-breakers are emotional; the others are physical or situational.

PHYSICAL FACTORS THAT CAN AFFECT SEXUAL FUNCTION

- Medications, such as antidepressants, mood stabilizers, contraceptive drugs, histamines, sedatives, antihypertensives, and/or medications for blood pressure or thyroid deficiency can decrease sexual desire.

- Fluctuating hormones.
- Midlife stress, including career change, relationships, loss, divorce, caring for parents, and financial concerns.
- Health issues, such as heart disease or diabetes.

Approximately 47 percent of women experience sexual difficulties according to the National Health and Social Life Survey and the Global Study of Sexual Attitudes and Behaviors, with a decrease of sexual desire being the most common.

IF YOUR LIBIDO IS DECLINING, ASK YOURSELF THESE QUESTIONS
1. Is it physical?
    *   Do you experience pain during intercourse?
    *   Can you achieve orgasm?
    *   Can you maintain arousal?
2. Is it lack of desire?
    *   Do you desire genital contact with your partner?
    *   Are you interested in sex, sexual thoughts, and fantasies?
3. Is it related to your relationship satisfaction?
    *   Are you happy with your relationship?
    *   Does your partner please you sexually?

Many aspects may affect your libido: desire, arousal, lack of lubrication, pleasure with orgasm, pain during intercourse, lack of sexual thoughts, aversion to sexual activity, sexual frequency, lack of receptivity, and relationship satisfaction. Medical conditions, such as depression, thyroid disease, androgen insufficiency, diabetes, cardiovascular disease or neurological disorders can also increase your risk of sexual dysfunction.

A variety of factors may affect sexual health: emotional, physical, medications, cultural, medical conditions, relationship satisfaction and midlife situations.

We live in a sexualized society that celebrates youth. This can leave a menopausal woman feeling frustrated and angry, self-conscious about her signs of aging, or scared about no longer being in the mood for sex. Many feel embarrassed to talk about it. We are sexual beings. Paying attention to your sexuality during menopause can deepen your relationship.

FIVE STEPS TO MANAGING A DECLINING LIBIDO
There is nothing worse than wanting to feel sexy and passionate with your lover, only to have your body and mind completely not the mood. Your sex life needs some tender loving care, and if you practice these five steps that sexy sizzle may return.

#1. Communication
If you are feeling undesirable and romance is no longer at the top of your list, the first thing you need to do is talk to your partner. As we get older, both men and women may notice a decline in their libido. It is normal for many to notice a change in sexual interest as we get older. Between the ages of 55 and 65, sexual desire may diminish for men and women. Having less sex is OK if both partners are satisfied with this change. If your partner is not OK with your declining libido, you need to address this symptom.

#2. Support

Getting support during this volatile time can strengthen your relationship, helping you emotionally and physically. It can be challenging to keep sexy feelings alive when you feel poorly about yourself and suffer from uncomfortable menopause symptoms. With some good old-fashioned support, trust, honesty, love, and commitment to get through it together, your relationship can soar to new heights.

How do you go about making this menopause miracle of love happen? First, you must acknowledge that your partner may be absolutely clueless about your menopause symptoms and emotional outbursts. While you are suffering from many changes both physical and emotional, you will also need to be at the helm educating your partner. This can be a difficult balancing act. Your partner must be informed so you can receive support.

The men I interviewed felt completely unprepared for their partner's menopausal transition. Most men survive their partner's monthly PMS and childbirth, but understanding these events will not necessarily give them the tools to cope with menopause. Unlike openly celebrated transitions like pregnancy, childbirth and child rearing, menopause is an occurrence in a woman's life that is still not openly discussed making it difficult for a man to understand and support his partner's transition.

Your partner may not be prepared to face the new reality of less sex, having to support you more, helping around the house, listening better, and turning on the air conditioning. He probably does not know what to do, or how to be around you during these unpredictable times. His greatest concern during your menopausal transition may be the fear of less sex. These worries are accelerated by his own fear of getting old and possibly by his own changes in sexual function. Understanding his fears will help the two of you communicate, so your partnership can be strengthened during menopause.

The majority of partners want to be supportive of their wives as they go through "the change," but you must let them know what you want. Do you need help around the house? Need a massage? A kiss? A snuggle? Do you want more cuddling and less sex? Need quiet time? Always remember that your partner has feelings too, so supporting him is also important. He should listen to your experience, and he has the right to express his feelings or opinions in return.

This open communication can bring you to a deeper level of intimacy, strengthening your relationship and making your passage smoother. Map a course, including a little humor, to ensure an easier route. If you forget where you put the keys and he is the one who usually forgets, have fun with it. Now it is his turn to "Go find the keys!" Or better yet, when you have hot flashes ask him to turn on the air conditioning and bring you a cool towel. Men love a mission. Make *you* his new mission, and make sure you reward him for pampering you.

If you are going through a seriously irritable stage, nothing makes you happy, and you are pissed off most of the time, give your partner warning. If he knows there is nothing he can do and you prefer to be alone, he can back off and give you space. Everyone will be happier. The more your partner knows about your experience, both emotionally and physically, the more he can show up for you as you need him. Ultimately, most guys want their women to be happy.

#3. Counseling

If you have a partner who does not support you, or is not willing to communicate, or if you yourself are struggling to communicate, it is time to seriously look at your relationship. Consider professional counseling.

#4. Adjust lovemaking activities

You may wish to consider new lovemaking activities. Allow more time for mental and manual stimulation. Remember the old days when you and your partner spent hours kissing and making love? Throw in a massage. Discuss sexual fantasies. Try a little afternoon delight in a new location; changing the time of day you engage in sexual activity and the location can add excitement. Reactivate the mind and heart. A little extra attention can reawaken a declining libido.

Sexual intercourse is not the only act in town. Oral sex is an intimate act that can allow you to have a great orgasm without the pain of sexual intercourse. You are entering a new world – be imaginative. Perhaps a new vibrating sex toy could be a fun companion. Add new sexual positions. Or "You show me and I'll show you," both learning something new about each other's pleasure. Feeling connected with your partner through the act of lovemaking can keep the passion alive, and help facilitate the return of your feeling sexy. A little effort can make all the difference in your sex life.

#5. Discuss options with your practitioner

If your fluctuating hormones are indeed affecting your libido, there are therapies available. See chapter 2 for more information.

LOW LIBIDO CHECKLIST

Discuss with your practitioner

• Sexual history • Life changes	• Relationship – are you still attracted to your partner? Are you in a healthy relationship?	• Medications • Health

---

HOW TO BOOST YOUR LIBIDO

If the flame of lust is still not burning after you have communicated with your partner, reached out for support, taken advantage of counseling, and adjusted lovemaking activities it may be time to discuss other options, both hormonal and non-hormonal, with your healthcare provider. A small adjustment can boost your libido.

ANDROGEN THERAPY

Many think androgens are a male hormone, but don't underestimate the power it has in a woman's body. Androgens are produced in the ovaries, adrenal glands and fat cells, and their role is to be converted to estrogen, as well as, stimulate sexual desire and help prevent bone loss.

It helps to think of androgen as a team comprised of hormone players. There are two primary androgens: testosterone and androstenedione, and a few co-players; DHT (dihydrotestosterone), DHEA (dehydroepiandrosterone), and DHEA-S (DHEA sulfate). If androgen levels are too high it can cause excessive hair growth (hirsutism), acne and thinning hair. Too little and you may feel fatigued and loose your sex drive.

Androgens decrease with age, and there is no sudden change during menopause. But by the time we reach menopause our androgen levels have declined 50 to 60 percent. The exception is surgical menopause. Androgen excess or deficiency is common during menopause and can create havoc on your well-being.

When women notice that their sex drive is diminishing, many of heard a dose of testosterone or dehydroepiandrosterone (DHEA) will fix the problem. The use of testosterone to treat a diminished libido is still controversial. The FDA has not approved testosterone therapies for women suffering from a declining libido, but there have been both preliminary scientific studies and extensive anecdotal reports that support the use of this therapy for improving the libido. Women who are on testosterone therapy should be monitored for increased lipids, excessive hair (hirsutism) and acne.

POSSIBLE TESTOSTERONE BENEFITS

- Increase energy levels
- Increase your sexual interest
- Enhances orgasm
- Increase bone density
- Give you a sense of well-being
- Help build lean muscle
- Helps deal with hot flashes
- Enhance short-term memory
- Increases skin elasticity

THE DOWNSIDE TO TESTOSTERONE THERAPY

* Increased cholesterol and unhealthy lipids
* Excessive facial or body hair
* Deeper voice
* Acne
* Weight gain
* Clitoral enlargement
* Changes in emotions, especially increased anger
* Being oversexed – no joke, it exists

Many pharmacies can custom-compound a preparation of transdermal micronized testosterone 2%(cream, ointment). A little compounded testosterone gel can be considered; but it has not been FDA-approved to treat a declining libido, and long-term safety data is lacking. As with all compounded formulations, there is no quality control in the preparation, and dosing may be inconsistent. Currently there are transdermal applications of testosterone in development (sprays, lotions and vaginal ring).

Estratest HS is a common estrogen-testosterone combination pill marketed in the USA, although it is technically only approved for hot flashes and not for sexual problems. In Canada, there is an oral testosterone off-label (not government approved) prescription drug used by women called Andriol (testosterone undecanoate).

The sophisticated orchestration of your hormones, your libido, and your relationship is complicated. Insist on good communication with both your clinician and partner. I personally discovered that my sex drive improved when I started hormone therapy.

THE TRUTH ABOUT DHEA

DHEA is another hormone in the androgen family. When you purchase DHEA, it is a dietary supplement, not a drug that is regulated by the government. It is often promoted as a libido-booster, an anti-aging supplement, an antidepressant, a memory aid, and a metabolism booster. DHEA is a promoted remedy for many health ailments, and has become a big seller at local health food stores. However, there is no scientific evidence supporting these claims. If your DHEA level is tested and shown to be below normal, then it may be reasonable to take a supplemental dose of DHEA 25 to 50 mg daily. However, if your DHEA is normal, then there is no reason to take DHEA as a supplement.

NON-HORMONAL THERAPIES TO TREAT A DECLINING LIBIDO

Going through menopause can be exhausting. Feeling good about yourself when everything is changing from your waistline to your sex life can be challenging. Often non-hormonal options may rescue a low libido and sizzle up your sex life. Many women suffer from vaginal dryness and using a sexual lubricant can be an immediate solution. Committing to new stress management practices like acupuncture, biofeedback, counseling, and some pampering time may reawaken your libido. Do not give up on your sex life.

SEX AND THE DREADED DRY VAGINA

The most common physical complaint during menopause is vaginal dryness. Needless to say, vaginal dryness does nothing for your libido! The good news is that vaginal dryness can be easily remedied. Bioadhesive lubricants, vaginal moisturizers, or estradiol vaginal creams are all excellent treatment options.

Suffering from vaginal dryness during lovemaking can add stress to a romantic relationship, zapping the sizzle out of your love life. Painful intercourse can quash even a healthy sex drive. Almost half of all women ages 40 to 65 complain of vaginal dryness; and one in five report painful intercourse. Vaginal estrogen cream or tablet used twice a week at a low dose has recently been approved by the FDA for the treatment of painful sex (dyspareunia).

Estrogen is the hormone that actually plumps up the cells in the vagina. When estrogen levels decline, the vaginal walls can become thinner, less elastic and dryer. Estrogen is important for maintaining vaginal health and lubrication. Sexual intercourse can actually tear the vaginal walls if not lubricated.

Bioadhesive lubricants such as Astroglide™ can be used for immediate relief, or Replens™, a vaginal moisturizer, applied twice a week. These options are found at most drug stores. The viscosity of a bioadhesive lubricant is thought to last longer than water-based gels. Lubrication can offer vaginal protection, as well as adding fun to your foreplay routine.

Other vaginal dryness options:

- Estradiol vaginal creams
- Estradiol vaginal tablets

If vaginal dryness is your only menopausal complaint, these local vaginal options can be taken without opposed progesterone therapy. If you have a host of other menopausal symptoms, including vaginal dryness, low-dose hormone therapy (pill, patch or gel) can likely bring relief.

Discuss your sexual concerns with your partner. There is nothing worse than lying in bed freaking out, feeling guilty and inadequate that your vagina is not lubricating as your partner is jumping through hoops to please you. Using lubricants or vaginal creams can help maintain your vaginal health and libido. Vaginal health can be remedied. Communicate with your partner about your physical and emotional sex concerns. Accept that your body is changing, and understand that options are available.

THE SECRET MEN DON'T WANT US TO KNOW

Men are worried their wives will no longer be interested in sex as they age and go through menopause, but a man's sexual life changes with age too! Men may start to notice a difference in erections. For some men, starting around the age of 40 they need more stimulation to get an erection.

I have had a number of girlfriends confess that their partners (after midlife) had a hard time getting erect; and when they did, it was a bit soft, did not last as long, the ejaculation was not forceful, and it took longer to reach orgasm. I was shocked at hearing this news!

Men go through physical and emotional changes too. Perhaps, witnessing our changes in sexuality is a reminder of their own deceleration. We may need a shot of lubrication, but our man could be facing sexual challenges he never expected. This will affect you too, so now is a good time to nurture a loving, sexual relationship. The communicating habits you create now will come in handy when your man begins to experience natural changes in his sexuality.

RELATIONSHIP REHAB

As if dealing with your partner weren't enough during an already overwhelming time in your life, what about the other people in your life? Just as you have to communicate with your partner, you may need to have heart-to-heart with other people in your life. It is unfortunate that our society does not prepare us, nor the ones we love, for menopause. There are no "hot flash seminars" or "cranky retreats" for menopausal gals.

THE GUY'S GUIDE TO UNDERSTANDING MENOPAUSE

There are a lot of different ways your partner can handle your menopause transition—some more helpful than others! If you are in a healthy relationship, most men will likely ask, "What can I do to help?" After all, when *you* are happy, *he* is happy. Men just want to know what *action* they need to take, so they can show up for you. Most do not want to buy a book and read about it-- you must tell them. They want to support you and survive your experience with as little effort and damage as possible.

On the next page is a survival list to share with your partner—it's like his menopause cheat sheet to use in case of emergency!

YOU...AND YOUR INNER SELF

As you develop a new relationship with yourself during menopause, you will have the wonderful opportunity to strengthen your current relationships, reconsider unhealthy relationships, and ultimately create the love you want in your life. You are at the helm of your relationships. Going through the menopause journey can stimulate internal growth, embracing a future with loving relationships. It can also instigate a little spring-cleaning in matters of the heart. Only you can determine if your "change" propels your life in a better direction. Women who have a loving relationship often have a smoother journey through menopause.

SURVIVAL TIPS FOR HIM

- Listen to her; don't criticize or try to fix her.
- Go with the flow; be prepared for constant mood swings.
- Be compassionate, and validate her experience (that means, agree with her).
- Tell your wife she can count on you.
- Cuddle more.
- Tell her she is beautiful.
- Appreciate her.
- Make time for the two of you.
- Keep romance alive.
- Surprise her with flowers for no reason at all.

- Understand her symptoms.
- Support her treatment choices.
- If she is resisting her own experience, encourage her to visit her doctor and develop a support team of girlfriends.
- Don't pursue sex if she is not in the mood; her body is changing.
- Don't think that her low libido or dry vagina is a reflection on your lovemaking skills.
- Don't ignore her hot flashes or night sweats. Offer to turn on the AC or buy her a little fan.
- If she's moody or cranky, offer support.

- As she is pigging out on junk food, don't tell her how fat she's getting. Really, don't.
- Surprise her with a date at the spa. Both of you can enjoy pampering.
- Tell her she is as beautiful as the day you met her. Let her know beauty isn't defined by age.
- If she's acting depressed, offer your support. Encourage her to seek professional help if she needs.
- If all else fails, disappear: step out for the afternoon or give her some space. Only after you have tried all the above tips.

SURVIVAL TIPS FOR EVERYONE ELSE

So what about everyone else? Friends, family, and co-workers need to survive your transition too.

- Inform your loved ones that you are going through changes emotionally and physically.
- Warn them if they notice changes from crankiness to depression, that you would appreciate some TLC.

- Invite them to support your self-esteem with compliments.
- Suggest that trying to fix you would not be a good strategy.

- Request lots of hugs.
- Encourage open communication.

MAKEOVER TIPS

* Communicate with your partner, so he or she understands your symptoms.
* Visit your clinician to discuss a declining libido and any issues with vaginal dryness.
* Don't let society make you feel inadequate about going through menopause.
* If you're libido is low, discuss your treatment options with your partner and practitioner.
* Communicate with loved ones and ask for support.
* Make time for romance with your partner; feeling connected during this time can make your transition smoother. Give yourself permission to spend the night cuddling if you are not "in the mood."
* Try new lovemaking routines with your partner; use a little creativity to spice up your sex life.
* Manage your menopause as a team. If your partner was there for you during childbirth, why not during menopause? Men love to solve-problems – let him be there for you. Use *The Guy's Guide to Understanding Menopause!*
* Purchase bioadhesive lubricant if you are suffering from vaginal dryness.
* Keep a sense of humor.
* Eat healthy, exercise and start loving your body during this powerful passage in your life.

GOOD NEWS: If They Run Away, They Can Always Run Back!

MAKEOVER TAKE ACTION LIST

- Buy bioadhesive lubricant or vaginal moisturizer if needed.

- Tape the "Survival Tips for Him" on your master bathroom mirror or his toolbox, so he can use it for quick reference in case of emergency. Having it in the bathroom offers privacy, and may open the door for conversation about your experience and his.

- Record relationship goals on page 192.

- Select one friend, family member or co-worker and share your current journey going through menopause; ask for support if you need it.

- If you are struggling with midlife issues, and your declining sex interest is the result of outside stress (divorce, empty nest, death of a family member, financial changes), schedule an appointment with a counselor.

IN YOUR ESSENTIAL PLANNER

- Schedule at least one night per week of intimacy time with your partner...or more, if interested, in Your Month-at-a-Glance Planner. You go, girl! If you don't use it, you may lose it!

- Record your feelings in your journal.

- Schedule an appointment with your healthcare provider to discuss your libido and any dry vagina symptoms – record doctor appointments in Your Month-at-a-Glance Planner.

- Document any changes in libido or vaginal dryness in your Medical Forms.

| Chapter 8 | Step Seven: Embracing Spirituality: What You Believe Can Change Your Experience |

When you feel like you have lost control of your health, beauty, relationships, career and purpose in life during the menopause journey, spirituality is sometimes the only thing left holding you up. How you choose to live life is often influenced by your spirituality. For one person, getting fired from a job seems like the ultimate tragedy. For another, it is an opportunity for growth. A lot depends on how you interpret events in your life. Your spiritual community can be an enormous source of support during menopause.

This chapter includes suggestions that can be applied to any spiritual belief system. Prayer, meditation and giving thanks can nourish your spirituality,bringing a new perspective your experience. Embracing spirituality during menopause can enrich your life and benefit your health.

WHAT YOU BELIEVE CAN CHANGE YOUR EXPERIENCE

The past six chapters have addressed serious physical aspects in the management of menopause. Yet I found that invisible thing we call spirituality to be one of the greatest sources of support during my passage through menopause. It is our nature as human beings to interpret the meaning and purpose of life. Thus, when we have a strong spiritual foundation, we have the ability to transcend many physical ailments. Being involved with a community that shares beliefs similar to your own can offer you support during menopause. It has been proven that people who have a strong sense of spirituality suffer less from hypertension, have better mental health, enjoy healthier lifestyles, and can actually live longer. Your spirituality can help define your menopause experience. Does menopause mean the loss of youth, beauty and childbearing years? Or does it represent a new beginning – focusing energy on your power to contribute to the community and personal growth?

Spirituality can mean different things to different people. In this chapter, I will refer to *spirituality* as the ultimate nature and purpose of our existence. Religions offer many people their source of spirituality. Others find it while enjoying a sunset, hiking or listening to music. Spirituality can offer hope and inner peace, profoundly affecting your physical and mental health and overall quality of life. Spirituality can be a wonderful tool, building good coping skills for managing stress, and offering a sense of well-being. The power of positive thinking can even prevent some health problems. Spirituality can be an asset to good health. What you believe can change your experience of menopause.

HOW MENOPAUSE CAN ENRICH YOUR SPIRITUALLY

Going through the menopause transition can stimulate growth – personal, physical and emotional. You are not only experiencing midlife changes (children moving out, relationships, finances, career, family and health), you are traveling through this transition with menopausal symptoms. Many women feel menopause represents the loss of fertility and youth. Suffering from feelings of loss and stress can make managing menopause more challenging.

It can be tough to redefine your purpose in life when you're enduring daily doses of hot flashes, dry itchy skin and an ever-expanding waistline. Menopause will force you to make choices. You can choose to view this time in your life as exciting and full of new possibilities. Or you can bitch about it and feel sorry for yourself.

I sat around complaining about each irritating symptom, gaining more and more weight as I stuffed my face with ice cream. Understandably, many ran away, leaving me isolated in the lowest emotional valley of my life. During this time, it was my spirituality that gave me the boost I needed to continue my climb up "Menopause Mountain." My spiritual journey changed my menopause experience. And balancing my hormones, switching to a good diet, and exercising daily sealed the deal. Marching through menopause forced me to ask myself some big life questions:

Who am I?

What do I need to be happy?

What are my passions, talents, and skills?

What is my purpose in life?

How do I contribute to society?

I was overwhelmed trying to answers these questions. After a few days squirming with this task, I developed a series of questions that took me on a spiritual path that helped me discover the answers for myself.

Find a quiet, comfortable place with paper and pen, clear your mind, breathe deeply, relax and let your inner self be expressed during this exercise. Just let the words and thoughts flow.

Who am I?

Name:

Gender and Age:

Family position in life (mother, daughter, grandmother, aunt, niece):

Career position in life:

Religion or Spiritual Preference:

How have you defined yourself through your life experiences? (Did you graduate college, marry, remain single, have children, travel, win a big contest, have an important event in your life that defined you?)

What makes you different than everyone else around you?

What are your wonderful qualities?

What are your less flattering qualities?

What is unique about you?

What do you value most in life?

How do you express yourself?

How do you think differently than others (do you see life through political eyes, do you see the positive or negative in life, do you always want to please people, do you naturally think things will work out or not?)

Are you are passionate about something special to you?

Study your answers. In one sentence answer, **who am I?**

What do I need to be happy?
List all the things you need to be happy in life – go for it here.

What are my passions, talents and skills?
List your talents/skills, everything you are naturally good at, and everything you are passionate about even if you are not good at it.

What is my purpose I life?
The answer to this question will help bring clarity to your daily life.
Why am I here?

Ask a close friend or family member what they think your purpose is in life.

How do I contribute to society?
Review all your answers above? Is there an area that defines you, brings you happiness, or that you excel at that you can share with others that will make a difference?

After answering these questions you may choose to set new life goals during your Menopause Makeover. Do you want to go back to work? Are you ready to retire? Would you like to volunteer at a favorite organization? Have you always wanted to do something but never had the time or courage to do? Start a new business? Go back to school? Learn a new language? Move to another location? Travel? Is it time to find new passions and give an unrealized dream attention?

Going through menopause can give you the opportunity for spiritual growth by redefining who you are, your purpose and what makes you happy; enabling you to develop new skills and passions; and determining how you want to contribute to society.

After answering the above question I had a better understanding of myself, with a new purpose no longer defined by youth and childbearing abilities, giving me something I had never felt before. Freedom. I now had the freedom to re-define myself. This can help you connect to your spirituality. Most of us have been so busy caring for others that we have had no time left to focus on our own powerful potential. It was exhilarating and liberating to focus on the *me* in menopause...*me*–no–pause. Having wandered away from my spiritual side as I became entangled in the confusion that accompanied menopause, eventually I discovered that menopause could enrich my spirituality!

My strong spiritual foundation helped me chart my way and successfully navigate the rough seas of miserable symptoms. The menopause/midlife combo is a wonderful opportunity to reinvent yourself, creating a life that embraces your uniqueness to contribute and make a difference. The expectation to reproduce is off your shoulders. Many people still believe it is an "end" once you reach menopause. The truth is, it is a new beginning to define your purpose outside of your biological ability to have children.

Menopause is also a perfect time to heal the past. Now is the time to address any unresolved feelings. In most religions and spiritual teachings, forgiveness can be an ingredient to help you move forward. If you are dealing with a complex situation, seek professional help. Attending to past hurts can set you free to build a life, painting a new future with a clean canvas.

Those of us going through the menopause journey have the incredible task of paving the way for our daughters. I have faith in the possibility that one day our society can fully accept this natural passage for a woman, and embrace it as a sacred event. How we interpret our menopause experience is the first step to that possibility. Tap into your spirituality to find your power and strength.

Where does your source of spirituality come from?

How can spirituality support your menopause experience?

THE POWER OF PRAYER AND MEDITATION

Can prayer and meditation equal good health? For thousands of years people have used prayer and/or mediation for health reasons, both for their own health, and the health of others. People have formed prayer groups to pray for someone's recovery. Others have mediated privately or in groups focusing on the health of an individual, group or the planet. There is research that claims meditation can decrease blood pressure, relax muscles, reduce oxygen intake, and lower stress hormones for hours after meditation.

Prayer and meditation have been a part of my life since childhood – sometimes a big part, sometimes less. With a Catholic upbringing I found comfort in the Lord's Prayer. When I grew up and traveled the world, I witnessed the beautiful aspects of other religions. Now I incorporate mediation as a tool to tap into my inner peace. I don't do either enough; but when I do pray or meditate, I feel grounded. Both prayer and meditation bring me serenity over my usually over-active mind. During menopause it can soothe many miserable symptoms from anxiety, to hot flashes to weight gain aggravated by stress hormones.

Millions and millions of people use prayer and meditation for health reasons.

DO SOMETHING KIND FOR SOMEONE, WITHOUT ANYONE FINDING OUT IT WAS YOU.

MIND-BODY BENEFITS OF MEDITATION

* Slows the progression of disease, and diminish stress.
* Lowers blood pressure.
* Reduces elevated cortisol levels caused by stress.

* Eases chronic pain.
* Relaxes muscles.
* Brings a sense of well-being.

Prayer and meditation can bring inner peace, resulting in a sense of freedom. Both prayer and meditation focus your attention away from the beehive of thoughts in your brain. These ancient practices help make people healthier and happier. Some claim that prayer and meditation can help extend life – slowing the effects of brain aging and improving memory. It has been proven that meditation practiced for a long period of time can actually alter brain-wave patterns. This can reduce stress levels, balance emotions and provide a sense of calm. During menopause this is an excellent prescription to help regain your health and build strong self-esteem.

HOW TO MEDITATE

- Find a comfortable, quiet spot where you can sit or lie down for at least 20 minutes uninterrupted (no music or phones).

- Adjust the temperature, so you are comfortable.

- Wear loose clothing.

- Set a timer for 20 minutes, so you don't obsess over time. Select a timer with a calming buzzer.

- Close your eyes halfway or in a relaxed closed position.

- If you sit, try to sit cross-legged with a straight back. If that is not possible, sit in a chair. If you lie down, open your arms and legs shoulder- and hip-width apart.

- Breathe through your nose, not your mouth.

- Breathe from your belly, not your chest.

- Take full, deep inhalations and exhale slowly.

- Relax your muscles.

- Don't have expectations. Be in the present moment.

- Many people use a personal mantra (a positive phrase declaring what you want to achieve) to meditate, or count their breaths (1 to 10, then repeat).

TRY THESE USEFUL PERSONAL MANTAS:

I am healthy.
I am strong.
I am loveable.
I honor my body.
May all be happy.
I have a happy marriage.
I am beautiful.
Abundance flows into my life.

- When your mind becomes busy with thoughts, refocus on your personal mantra, or breaths (you can also use a phrase from the Menopause Prayer or A Woman's Prayer on pages 144 and 145).

- Do not meditate after a meal, or you may fall asleep.

- After you have trained your mind to focus on your mantra, or counting of breaths, begin to focus on nothing at all! True silence of the mind is the ultimate goal.

- Meditation requires patience. It is OK to have "monkey brain" (busy thinking) sometimes; mastering this is a normal part of the meditation practice.

PRAYERS

Feeling vulnerable and lonely during my menopause journey, I searched for an inspiring prayer. Not being able to find one I liked, I decided to write my own prayer to help give me strength during this transition.

An interesting thing happened when I began to write my personal menopause prayer – the words flew onto my computer screen as if something bigger than myself was creating this prayer. Twenty minutes later I not only had the prayer I needed, but I had two prayers. These prayers helped me in my darkest menopause times. When I read them in silence or out loud, I felt strength and hope that I would get through menopause a better person.

No matter what your spiritual preference is, as women we often find comfort and peace in words. You can call these words a prayer, poem, short story, or a mantra. Being brought up Catholic, I find comfort in the word *Lord*. To me the Lord is something bigger than me, yet the Lord also refers to that something special deep inside. Whatever your spiritual practice feel free to use one or both prayers. You may wish to omit the word *Lord* in *A Woman's Prayer* if that makes you feel more connected to the message. Honor your spiritual path.

Now, I share my menopause prayers with you. I hope you find comfort in them too.

MENOPAUSE PRAYER

Give me strength to see the beauty in womanhood to embrace my passage from the giving of life to the giving of myself.

Show me my special purpose, releasing my spirit from expectations.

Open my heart to love, so I may nourish my soul.

Bring light into my darkness, so I may see that you shine eternally.

Hold my hand, so I am not alone.

Give me hope to see a bright future.

Shower me with patience to understand.

Wrap me with courage to celebrate my choices.

Shelter me from fear. Help me honor my body.

Quiet my raging emotions. Cool my ever-changing body temperature. Steady me with your strength.

Lift me up to see beauty in my life, not in my face.

Remind me that I am desirable.

Empower me to see the good in everyone.

Open my eyes to appreciate my abundance.

Set my spirit free, so I may find my true calling.

Watch over me, so my soul may flourish.

May I find a sanctuary in your everlasting love.

A WOMAN'S PRAYER

Lord grant me:

Serenity to accept my changes

Power to focus on the positive

Trust that I will receive support

Harmony in my emerging self

Lord grant me:

Self-acceptance in my beauty

Abundance of love

Freedom to dream

Balance to honor myself

Lord grant me:

Healing to resolve the past

The ability to manifest new beginnings

The strength to surrender

Moments to celebrate

Lord grant me:

Courage to forgive

Gratefulness for my gifts

Patience to understand that "change" is a blessing wrapped in your love.

Just as I wrote these prayers to help me through tough menopausal times, you too may wish to write your own prayer. It is very therapeutic.

HOW TO WRITE A PERSONAL MENOPAUSE PRAYER

- Find a quiet room.
- Make sure there are no distractions.
- Sit down with pen and paper or in front of your computer.
- Clear your mind.
- Let go of your expectations.
- Close your eyes to connect with your inner self.
- Take a few deep breaths.
- Ask yourself, "What wisdom do I need to receive today?"

- Just start writing/typing.
- Let the words flow—don't judge yourself.
- It's OK to cry during this experience. You are giving your spirit a place to be expressed.
- When the words stop flowing, read your prayer.
- Refer to this prayer when you feel lonely, sad, frustrated, angry or lost.

CELEBRATE THE CHANGE

Now that your spiritual energy is flowing, let's harness that power so you can go through "the change" celebrated! Why is it we celebrate childbirth despite the physical pain? Why do we celebrate a wedding even though it usually causes great stress? Society has taught us to look at these transitions in life as a celebration, whether they were pleasant or not. Perhaps as a way to bring order to civilization, or to bring a sense of peace, so people could find joy in the changes of life. Knowing this little fact of life, let's ask ourselves, "why can't we go through menopause celebrated too?" The answer: We can! We can change the way society views menopause when *we* decide to celebrate our transition. If we continue to cling to youth, we cannot embrace the wisdom of aging. So how do we go through "the change" celebrated? We *choose* to go through "the change" celebrated! We must practice this celebration daily, despite frustrating symptoms and challenging midlife changes. It is your choice. If you look at menopause as a passage to be celebrated, so will others.

HOW TO CELEBRATE MENOPAUSE

- Write 3 reasons to celebrate menopause (come on now, I know you can find a few reasons).

- Read this list everyday—once in the morning, and once before going to bed.

- Pray of meditate every day for support to be strong during this transition, because on the other side of menopause are new possibilities.

- Tell your loved ones and friends that you have made a choice to celebrate your passage.

- Think about this passage in your life as a positive experience.

- Embrace the many stages of womanhood. Each stage is a contribution to humankind.

- Pamper yourself—you are celebrating the new you.

MAKEOVER TIPS:

- Nurture your spirituality. Read, pray, meditate, go on a spiritual retreat.

- Take care of your body. Be still, get rest and make time for pampering.

- Expand your mind. Join a spiritual group; read new books and articles.

- Look at your career or consider working/volunteering again. Find situations that can bring you joy. Start your own business. Write a book. Finish that scrapbook you started years ago.

- Go back to school. Do you have unrealized dreams? Are you curious to learn something new? Find a new passion.

- Travel. Visit the places in your dreams.

- Start a diary focusing on what you feel, not what you do.

- Make time every day to practice your spirituality. Pray, meditate, read, join support groups, volunteer, take a walk, attend spiritual services, enjoy quiet time.

- Remember to laugh.

- Choose to spend time with those with whom you share a healthy relationship.

MAKEOVER TAKE ACTION LIST

* Record your spiritual goals on page 193.
* Nourish spirituality in your life.
* Add prayer and/or meditation to your daily routine.
* Answer the "big" questions on page 137.
* In a peaceful setting, read aloud the *Menopause Prayer* or *A Woman's Prayer* at least once a week.
* Write your own personal menopause prayer.
* Twice a day say, "I have a choice to go through 'the change' celebrated."
* Schedule time so you may embrace spirituality daily.

IN YOUR ESSENTIAL PLANNER

* Add daily spiritual goals to your Month-at-a-glance Planner.
* Write daily in your journal.

	Step Eight: Creating Happiness
Chapter 9	How to Be Happy During "The Change"

Was I happy about going through menopause? Was I happy about miserable menopause symptoms? Was I happy getting fat and cranky? Was I happy living with hot flashes? Was I happy living with the air conditioner on full-blast in the winter? Was I happy? *Happy?* What was there to be happy about? I was miserable and pissed off that everything in my life was changing. I had to change my blouse after every hot flash. I had to change the way I ate. I had to change the way I took care of my skin. I had to change the way I had sex with my husband. Everything was changing, and I was not happy about it. How does anyone find happiness going through all this physical and emotional change?

Webster's New World Dictionary defines happiness as "a feeling of pleasure, contentment or joy." This can be very difficult to achieve during the menopause journey. An avalanche of miserable symptoms and midlife changes can cover any hope of feeling happy.

This section is dedicated to digging out those happy feelings, and unearthing coping skills to restore balance and joy. Once you embrace change, happiness is possible.

HOW HAPPY ARE YOU?

You would think answering this question would be easy, but it's more complicated than you might think. Imagine happiness like a pie made up of many slices like health, career, self-esteem and relationships. . When each slice of the pie is full and intact, the entire happiness pie is complete and you will feel fulfilled. If any one piece of the pie is missing, it will affect the pie as a whole: if your health is failing, your ability to work could be comprised; if you don't have a strong self-esteem, your love life may suffer; if money is missing in your life, your health and self-esteem may deteriorate. When we find a balance in all areas of our life, happiness is almost always guaranteed.

So, are you happy? Let's rate the different areas of your life. Be honest – the only way to grow happier is to recognize those areas that you need to work on. This is a great opportunity to achieve high levels of happiness. Only when you're happy, will you be able to live to your full potential.

HAPPINESS QUESTIONNAIRE

Rate each category 1 to 10 – number 10 being over-the-moon happy, number 1 being not happy at all.

☐ Health		☐ Relatives	
☐ Love (with someone special)		☐ Children	
☐ Spirituality		☐ Home	
☐ Self-esteem		☐ Travel/adventure	
☐ Work		☐ Education/learning	
☐ Money (do you feel safe)		☐ Neighborhood	
☐ Hobbies		☐ Giving	
☐ Friends		☐ Creativity	

SCORE RESULTS:

128-160 You are living life to the fullest, embracing the positive. You are creating your world from a place of love and joy. Start sharing your secret with others!

96-127 You have successfully focused on some aspects of your life, but are not living in balance with others. Direct your attention with intention to one new area per week. Set goals to grow, and be open to possibilities within the areas of your life that are not yet satisfying. Continue to foster the areas giving you pleasure. Give thanks for all that you have.

64-95	You are below average on the happiness scale. Ask yourself what's keeping you from being as happy as possible. Make a list of things in your life that cause you unhappiness. Are there solutions? If you cannot find resolution to these areas, ask for help – personal or professional. Look at the areas of your life that bring happiness. Can you create positive change? Accept and love yourself.
32-63	You probably have situations in your life that are keeping you from being happy. How can you achieve happiness in the areas you can control? Make a list of the things that make you happy. Nourish these areas. In the areas that seem hopeless, reach out for help. Visualize happiness in all areas of your life. Pray or meditate for happiness and gratitude. Embrace your potential in all areas of your life.
0-31	You may not feel happiness is achievable, or may not have learned skills to be happy. Start seeing the positive in your life. Take control of areas that appear hopeless. Appreciate the few things in your life that bring you joy. Build on those areas. Once your happiness level grows, expand to other areas. *Decide* to be happy. Happiness needs to be nourished.

How do you feel about your level of happiness? What's incredible about this process is that life is always changing, so your level of happiness will change too.

I do this exercise every New Year's Eve. Five years ago I had a great career, but no love. After looking at this situation, it dawned on me that I was working long hours so I had no time for love. After finding a balance in these two areas, I now have a great love and a new career I love, too! I focused on the area that was not fulfilled and took action. I had to look at the whole picture so I could make change. Consider these questions:

* What areas need attention in your life?
* Is there a pattern of areas that are not fulfilled and areas that are making you deliriously happy?
* Is there an action you can take to initiate positive change?

HOW TO CREATE HAPPINESS

Menopause will force you to look at all areas of your life. You may start with the physical dealing with hot flashes and weight gain, but if you don't look at your whole picture, you won't have the tools to achieve happiness.

You can create happiness. Even out of great tragedy, the human spirit is capable of achieving happiness. Do you want to be happy? Believe it or not, it is *your* choice.

STEPS TO CREATING HAPPINESS

- Decide to be happy. Happiness is a choice.

- Relax and laugh more often. When you start to feel stressed, breathe deep—try not to worry so much.

- Understand that happiness is not a full-time job.

- Find lessons in the challenges of life. What can you learn from a difficult situation? If you can take away a life lesson from a challenging situation, it is easier to get past negative feelings so you can be happy.

- Live in the present. You cannot fix the past and do not know the future. Embrace the now.

- Be grateful for the many gifts in your life.

- Accept yourself—remember the "perfect you" inside.

- Be a positive thinker.

- Create goals that bring you joy.

- Focus on the journey, not the payoff.

- Visualize your dreams.

- Nourish healthy relationships in your life.

- Spoil your body. Pamper yourself. Eat well and exercise.

- Give back to others.

- Avoid smoking, drugs or excessive alcohol.

- Journal

RESPECT YOUR BODY – IT IS THE PATH TO YOUR SPIRIT.

Happiness Journaling Exercise

One of the strongest tools for personal growth is journaling. It is a safe place for expression. The process of writing allows you to analyze and contemplate your life. It is also a wonderful tool to sort out thoughts and feelings. Journaling can offer you healing, the opportunity to solve problems, awaken your spirit and strengthen your inner voice. Recording your feelings can offer you a new perspective and help you achieve balance in your life.

Find a special notebook, diary, or journal and select a writing pen just for journaling. You can journal when you first wake up or some people prefer to journal in the quiet hours before bedtime. Whether you choose to journaling in the morning or evening, journal daily.

Answer these questions before starting your journal – your answers will be a great springboard for you to start journaling.

What is your definition of happiness?

What things made you happy in your past?

What makes you happy now?

What areas from the Happiness Questionnaire need focus to create happiness?

Set goals in areas that you can improve.

Every day, write what you will do to make yourself happy,
and how you will make others happy.

◇◇◇

SURROUND YOURSELF WITH POSITIVE PEOPLE.

◇◇◇

MANIFEST HAPPINESS: KEEP YOUR LIFE SIMPLE

You need space and clarity to create happiness. Simplifying your life—from your home to your schedule—can help create that space in your life. If your home is cluttered, clean up your space. Clutter is like a self-imposed fat suit – stop hiding under a mess. Get to the root of your cluttered life. Are you messy because you are lazy – how can a lazy person grow? Are you living in clutter to hide your disappointment in life – you cannot overcome disappointment by hiding from the truth. Clutter is a symptom of something not working in your life. This manifestation may hold you back from happiness.

If your to-do list is jam-packed every day, focus on tasks that make your life better and make you feel happy. We all have to shop for food, pay bills, and do laundry. Spread your life's duties throughout the week, so each day has free time scheduled for you. When you have the burden of chores or tasks weighing on your spirit, you cannot grow. Like throwing a brick on a plant – it cannot grow and shine squashed under the brick. Lift the brick of too many chores or tasks that can be managed over time. Manage your life, honoring that you are the number one priority. Sometimes you may have to say no– you don't have to do everything for everyone. Focus on you.

MAKEOVER TIPS:

* Make time for yourself
* Remember that you don't have to say "yes" to everything
* Simplify your life
* Delegate—you don't have to do everything on your own
* De-clutter your house
* Have a good attitude
* Set small, attainable goals
* Reward your progress
* Share your goals with loved ones, so you are accountable

SIMPLIFY YOUR LIFE.

A GOOD ATTITUDE OPENS THE DOOR TO HAPPINESS

Have you noticed that cranky crabby people are usually not happy people? No matter what your life situation, having a good attitude can open the door to your happiness. What exactly is a good attitude? It has to do with how you interpret your current situation. Being optimistic allows you to attract good situations and good people into your life. A good attitude can actually improve your stress levels and health. By practicing a hopeful outlook, you are telling yourself and the world that you believe good things come your way. When you are negative, that pessimistic outlook can actually attract bad results. Usually fear fuels negativity. If you start having a bad attitude ask yourself, "What am I afraid of?" What is the underlying fear behind this negative attitude? Practice saying to yourself everyday, "No matter what happens today, I will see the good."

POSITIVE THOUGHTS + POSITIVE ACTION = GOOD ATTITUDE

THE MENOPAUSE MAKEOVER HAPPINESS FORMULA

* Empower yourself to embrace change.
* Accept change; it is the only constant in life.
* If you have the courage to change, happiness is your choice.
* Acknowledge your possibilities.
* Give thanks for what you have.
* Live in the present, so you can witness happiness.

HOW TO GET WHAT YOU WANT IN LIFE

After evaluating happiness in your life, you may be asking, "So, what do I want in life, and how do I get it?" As women, we often focus our attention on what other people want, and we try to make sure they get it. Often we have no idea what makes us happy, other than being with the people we love. Many women arrive at the menopause transition completely clueless as to what makes them happy or what they want out of life.

Examine areas in your life denying you personal fulfillment; the Happiness Questionnaire can give you a head start. Setting goals is one of the simplest, most effective ways to create change and navigate the path toward happiness. These journal exercises can be very motivating. Once you identify your goals, you will be able to track results (more on goal-setting in Chapter 12) to build self-confidence.

GOAL-SETTING EXERCISE

Forms for these goal-setting exercises can be found in Chapter 12.

* List everything you have ever wanted to do in your lifetime. How can you start turning these dreams into realities?

* Make a list from the Happiness Questionnaire starting with the lowest score. Next to each area, jot down what you can do to add happiness to that area.

* Each week, go down that list and start incorporating an "action" you can do to improve these areas.

* Set short-term and long-term goals. Set daily, monthly, 6-month, 1-year and 5-year goals. Refer to your list daily. Visualize reaching your goals.

* Set realistic goals.

* Be clear and concise in your goal setting. For example: I want to travel and see the world (a vague goal). A more concise goal: I want to see Italy, Spain and Greece by the end of next year (a focused, achievable goal). If money is an issue, set a goal to raise money or get a small weekend job – and start saving.

* Update your goals. When a new desire comes up, add it to the list.

* Prioritize your goals.

* Have small and large goals. You will reach some faster than others. Some may be complex and need more time.

* Every day, record your actions toward obtaining your goals.

ONCE YOU BEGIN SEEING RESULTS, REWARD YOURSELF. CELEBRATE. CREATING A LIFE YOU WANT TO LIVE IS A POWERFUL TOOL TO LIVING JOYFULLY.

GRATITUDE

Using the power of gratitude is one of the easiest ways to create happiness in your life. We often go through our busy days without acknowledging the wonderful gifts that surround us. Appreciating these blessings will create a positive attitude, that will in turn attracting happiness and abundance. People who are grateful often have better health and experience less stress. By practicing gratitude, you can increase your self-esteem and energy.

Often we resist events or people in our lives. This negative energy will assure only negative outcomes. Gratitude is a positive energy, attracting positive results. You will attract whatever energy you send out. It is easy to get caught up in being negative and angry when life does not go the way we want it. To break this destructive behavior, start examining your life and give thanks for all that is positive. Accept people or situations for what they are, this helps eliminate resistance in life. When you conquer resistance, you will attract happiness.

ACCEPTANCE + GRATITUDE = HAPPINESS

Gratitude exercise

- Mentally make a list of all the things you feel grateful for. Sometimes you can find gratitude during prayer or a meditation session focused on thankfulness.
- List 10 things you are grateful for:

1.

2.

3.

4.

5.

6.

7.

8.

9.

10.

* Let people know how special they are to you, and how thankful you are that they are in your life.
* When something negative happens, try to find the positive in it. Is there something to be thankful for in that experience?

◇◇

HAPPINESS IS A CHOICE.

◇◇

MAKEOVER TIPS

* Be aware and grateful for the good things in your life.
* Practice forgiveness.
* Focus your attention on happiness and positive thinking.

MAKEOVER TAKE ACTION LIST

* Reflect on your answers from the Happiness Questionnaire. In what areas can you increase your happiness? Set achievable goals of yourself.
* Complete the happiness journaling exercise on page 153.
* De-clutter and simplify your life.
* Have a good attitude everyday.
* Read The Menopause Makeover Happiness Formula once a week.
* Complete the goal-setting journaling exercise on pages 187 to 199.
* Complete the gratitude exercise on page 157.
* Discuss your goals with loved ones.
* Show appreciation for the people and things in your life.
* Be *happy*, you are about to begin your *Menopause Makeover*!

IN YOUR ESSENTIAL PLANNER

* Set happiness goals in Your Month-at-a-Glance Planner.
* Make a list of the things that make you happy and record in Your Journal.
* Acknowledge people/things in your life daily in your 12-Week Plan.
* List things you are grateful for Your Gratitude List.
* Add a list of friends who you feel happy around to Your Menopause Makeover Contacts.

PART 2

Your Menopause Makeover:
Planning Your Transformation

Chapter 10	Getting the Facts Straight: The 10 Facts You Need to Know to Be Successful

In Part Two, all the pieces of the puzzle come together to create the new you. You can personalize your *Menopause Makeover* in three easy steps.

1. Identify the facts and tools needed to begin your Makeover.
2. Create your health profile.
3. Set goals for your 12-week makeover.

After completing these three steps, you are ready to begin The Menopause Makeover 12-Week Plan!

THE TEN MENOPAUSE MAKEOVER FACTS

Identify the facts and tools needed to begin your Makeover. To successfully set achievable goals, track your progress and stay motivated, you need to take stock of your current situation. In order to take eight Menopause Makeover steps forward, you need to know where you stand.

THE TEN FACTS

FACT #1: You have to get real to make change
FACT #2: The Numbers don't lie: the BMI Chart
FACT #3: You have an ideal weight unique only to you
FACT #4: Knowing your numbers can save your life: The Waist-Hip Ratio

Fact #5:	Change is all about balance: body fat and lean body mass
Fact #6:	Counting calories matters: what you put in your mouth can change your health
Fact #7:	Burning calories matters: the Basal Metabolic Rate (BMR)
Fact #8:	You gotta move to get anywhere! Exercise and physical activity can move you into a healthy future
Fact #9:	It takes energy to process food: the thermic effect of food
Fact #10:	You Must Commit to the MENOPAUSE MAKEOVER FOOD PYRAMID

FACT #1: YOU HAVE TO GET REAL TO MAKE CHANGE

Before you can set goals, you must get real with yourself. Whether you are addressing hot flashes or weight gain, or just trying to eat healthy and include exercise in your daily routine, understanding your physical statistics will give you the opportunity to set attainable goals. Do you know your ideal weight? What percent of your body weight is fat? How many calories do you need to maintain your current weight? What daily calorie intake will smooth the progress of achieving your perfect weight?

By getting real with yourself and facing the facts, you will increase your odds of accomplishing your Menopause Makeover goals successfully.

FACT #2: THE NUMBERS DON'T LIE: THE BMI CHART

One of the most common charts used for determining body fatness is the *BMI* Chart. BMI stands for "body mass index." The BMI calculation is a measurement of your body fat composition that uses a mathematical formula: your weight in kilograms divided by your height in meters squared (BMI=kg/m2). Don't be intimidated by the math! The math has already been taking care of, so all you have to do is check the BMI chart to easily get your body fat calculation. All you need to know is your height and current weight.

More than one third of adults in the United States are overweight or obese. Many health-care providers use the BMI Chart as a gauge to monitor weight because it is inexpensive and easy-to-use. Being overweight can lead to serious health problems such as heart disease, diabetes and cancer. In Chapter 11, I'll walk you through the process of determining your BMI. If your result is 18.5 to 24.0, you are within "normal" range. If your result is 25 to 29.9, you are overweight; 30 and above, you are obese.

The BMI Chart is a great tool, but it does not account for your body composition. If you are muscle-bound (muscle weighs more than fat), your BMI Chart results may categorize you as obese when, in fact, you are healthy. If you are over 50 years of age with a lesser amount of amount of muscle mass, the BMI Chart may underestimate your weight. If you are muscle bound or have a lesser amount of muscle mass and over the age of 50, you may wish to use the lean body weight formula in Chapter 11 for a more accurate calculation.

FACT #3: YOU HAVE AN IDEAL WEIGHT UNIQUE ONLY TO YOU

Many skinny celebrities we see on television spend a lot of time maintaining those slender silhouettes. From my work as a producer, I know firsthand some of the challenges that celebrities experience while attempting to maintain their girlish figures. A famous friend of mine is short and square in build. She will never have that tall, lean, skinny look. It is not her body type. Yet she is very healthy – she eats well, exercises daily, and she looks great! She honors her ideal weight.

In Chapter 11 we will calculate your healthy weight, so you can begin accepting your perfect size. Do not be influenced by the media's interpretation of beauty. Everybody is different! Your frame, bone structure and body composition are unique to you.

FACT #4: KNOWING YOUR PROPORTIONS CAN SAVE YOUR LIFE: THE WAIST-HIP RATIO

The BMI chart is a good weight gauge. Where we hold our fat – hips or belly – can indicate our health risks. Women with pear-shaped bodies, who carry their weight on the hips, have a lower risk for health issues such as coronary heart disease, diabetes, blood pressure and obesity. Women who carry the majority of their weight around the middle, the "apple" body shape, have a higher risk for health concerns. A waist-hip ratio above 0.85 puts you at risk. For women with apple body shapes, it is important to keep excess fat off that midsection. This is a true challenge during menopause. My menopause fat was lumped in the middle, putting me in the unhealthy category! It took hard work to reduce that menopause midsection. You will measure your waist and hips to determine your hip-to-waist ratio in Chapter 11.

FACT #5: CHANGE IS ALL ABOUT BALANCE: BODY FAT AND LEAN BODY MASS

After you determine your BMI, we will calculate how much body fat and lean body mass (muscles, organs, bones) you have. This exercise will show you how much fat your body is carrying. During menopause, fat shifts to the midsection, so you will determine both your body fat and lean body mass in the next chapter. Remember, you can turn fat into muscle. After I initially calculated my lean body mass and body fat (a whopping 38 percent!), I became committed to a daily exercise routine. I was determined to turn that fat back into muscle! Knowing exactly how much fat and lean body mass you have will allow you to set goals you can track. Build muscle; it will burn fat! You will be stronger and feel better.

FACT #6: COUNTING CALORIES MATTERS

A calorie is a unit of energy, a measurement. It is the amount of energy it takes to raise the temperature of 1 gram of water 1.8 degrees Fahrenheit. You can consume calories and burn calories. For many of us, a calorie is a pain in the butt – or a pound on our menopausal midsection. As discussed in Chapter 3, counting calories can change your health profile. As we age and lose muscle mass, we need fewer calories to survive. Knowing how many calories you need to consume in order to maintain, lose or add weight is an important step during The Menopause Makeover. Whether you are a vegetarian or meat-lover, the number of calories you consume and burn each day will affect your health.

One pound of fat equals 3500 calories. Consuming 500 fewer calories per day for one week equals one pound of fat. In the next chapter, you will calculate your current calorie consumption and calorie needs. Then you will use this number to manage you food intake and physical activity during the 12-Week Menopause Makeover. Using your food planner template located in the Chapter 13 will give you the tools to stay on track with your calorie goal.

FACT #7: BURNING CALORIES MATTERS: THE BASAL METABOLIC RATE (BMR)

The minimum calories needed to keep you alive (heartbeat, breathing) while you are asleep is called basal metabolic rate (BMR). It is the smallest amount of energy burned by the body in a resting state. Your BMR number can be used to calculate the speed of your metabolism, the rate your body burns calories, so you can determine how many calories you need to maintain, lose or increase your weight.

Both genetics and environment can determine your BMR. For example, some people are born with a high metabolism. Men have more muscle mass, so their metabolism is higher than a woman's. Your BMR lowers as you age. These are all factors you cannot change.

Your weight and body fat percentage both affect BMR. These factors *can* be changed. Exercise can raise your BMR; and exercise creates muscles, increasing BMR.

Your Basal Metabolic Rate is the largest factor (60-70 percent) in your total calorie expenditure. Calculating your BMR is the first part of the equation used in determining how many calories your body requires at its current weight. In the next chapter, you'll calculate your BMR to figure out your caloric needs for your Menopause Makeover.

FACT #8: YOU GOTTA MOVE TO GET ANYWHERE!

The second factor in your total calorie expenditure (20-30 %) is how much energy your body expends during physical activity. Refer to the Calories Burned Per Hour chart, Chapter 4 to calculate your energy expended during physical activity. Consider adding a few new activities to your daily routine.

FACT #9: IT TAKES ENERGY TO PROCESS FOOD

The third factor in your total calorie expenditure is the thermic effect of food. Thermic effect of food is the amount of energy it takes your body to digest food. It takes your body more energy to process protein over fat, with carbohydrates falling in the middle. Why does this matter for your makeover? Knowing what foods speed up your metabolism can help you lose weight. Exercise can also speed up your metabolism, as discussed in Chapter 4. When you eat foods that can speed up your metabolism combined with exercise, you have a winning formula. More good news, while you are sleeping, resting and eating your body is also burning energy.

FACT #10: YOU MUST COMMIT TO THE MENOPAUSE MAKEOVER FOOD PYRAMID

It is important to fuel your body with proper nutrients daily. Eating a properly balanced meal three times per day, along with two to three snacks, will ensure that your metabolism stays active, your body is nourished and you maintain a healthy weight for your Menopause Makeover. The Menopause Makeover Food Pyramid provides you with the correct proportions of calories from protein, carbohydrates, and fats—exactly what your body needs to be healthy during menopause! See Chapter 3 for more information.

The Menopause Makeover Food Pyramid

25% of calories from healthy fats

35% of calories from low-fat, lean protein

40% of calories from low- to medium-glycemic carbs

MAKEOVER TIPS

Don't skip the next chapter. Chapter 11 will help you craft your personal caloric needs and weight-loss goals. It is one of the most important chapters in this book! Without your starting numbers, you have no reference point for setting and tracking goals.

MAKEOVER TAKE ACTION LIST

* Purchase a fabric tape measure to be used in Chapter 11.
* Make sure you have a calibrated scale.
* Make a copy of The Menopause Makeover Food Pyramid located on page 52 and tape it to your refrigerator.

ONCE YOU FOCUS ON WHAT YOU WANT, YOU HAVE TO BELIEVE WITH ALL YOUR HEART THAT IT IS POSSIBLE.

Chapter 11	Putting it All Together Doing the Math is an Equation for Success

As my waistline was rapidly expanding, I finally had to admit that my health and beauty were quickly declining. Menopause had become a runaway train, and I was tied to the tracks of my youthful past.

When I created the menopause makeover I decided to take a "before" photograph in my favorite swimsuit and take measurements, so I would have a reference point to set goals. I was too embarrassed to ask my husband to take the "before" photograph for fear he would regret marrying me, so I secretly packed my swimsuit, grabbed a tripod along with the family digital camera, and took a self-portrait body shot in my office. What happened next shook my world. When I downloaded my bikini pictures I was horrified - I was fat! My favorite swimsuit was stretched over my hips like I had squeezed into a child's swimsuit. Sobbing like someone died, I feared I would never return to my healthy sexy self again. To add salt to the wound as I was downing a chocolate covered donut, I took out the tape measure and documented my sorry statistics.

An hour passed of feeling hopeless, old and ugly staring at this new depressing evidence. Then something interesting happened. Knowing the awful truth was actually liberating. There was no more avoiding the hard fact that going through menopause completely changed my body shape, skin, moods and outlook on life - and not for the good. I asked myself, "Do I give up and let this transition get the best of me, or do I arm myself with information and take action?"

After I reviewed my statistics and looked at the hideous photograph, I decided I needed some inspiration. I found a photograph of a healthy me taken a few years earlier for inspiration (you can see those photographs in the Introduction). Next I did some calculations so I knew what healthy was for my size, then set obtainable goals. Those terrifying measurements actually kicked me in the butt to make change.

In this chapter you will do some math--don't worry, the formulas are easy!--to take stock your current health profile and determine your personal makeover goals. You will record your statistics and find a photograph taken of you in the past when you felt good about yourself to use as inspiration for your makeover.

You may feel resistance to this part of your Menopause Makeover. Who among us is friends with a tape measure and likes math? But it is this part of your makeover that will reflect the truth about your health profile. Understanding your personal statistics will allow you to face your demons. Once you set goals that can change your health, your demons will crumple under the sword of knowledge. You will have power over your life again. Doing the math is an equation for success!

CREATE YOUR HEALTH PROFILE

This chapter is the second step needed to begin your Menopause Makeover. It includes all of the calculations you will use in when you create your personal menopause makeover in the Essential Planner. You'll reference this chapter throughout the 12-Week Plan.

CALCULATE YOUR BODY MASS INDEX

Calculate your body mass index using the BMI chart.

Locate your height at the top of this chart, and weight on the left side. Determine your current Body Mass Index.

My BMI is: _____

Body Mass Index (BMI) Chart

BMI	19	20	21	22	23	24	25	26	27	28	29	30	31	32	33	34	35
Height								**Weight (in Pounds)**									
4"10"	91	96	100	105	110	115	119	124	129	134	138	143	148	153	158	162	167
4"11"	94	99	104	109	114	119	124	128	133	138	143	148	153	158	163	168	173
5'	97	102	107	112	118	123	128	133	138	143	148	153	158	163	168	174	179
5'1"	100	106	111	116	122	127	132	137	143	148	153	158	164	169	174	180	185
5'2"	104	109	115	120	126	131	136	142	147	153	158	164	169	175	180	186	191
5'3"	107	113	118	124	130	135	141	146	152	158	163	169	175	180	186	191	197
5'4"	110	116	122	128	134	140	145	151	157	163	169	174	180	186	192	197	204
5'5"	114	120	126	132	138	144	150	156	162	168	174	180	186	192	*198	204	210
5'6"	118	124	130	136	142	148	155	161	167	173	179	186	192	198	204	210	216
5'7"	121	127	134	140	146	153	159	166	172	178	185	191	198	204	211	217	223
5'8"	125	131	138	144	151	158	164	171	177	184	190	197	203	210	216	223	230
5'9"	128	135	142	149	155	162	169	176	182	189	196	203	209	216	223	230	236
5'10"	132	139	146	153	160	167	174	181	188	195	202	209	216	222	229	236	243
5'11"	136	143	150	157	165	172	179	186	193	200	208	215	222	229	236	243	250
6'	140	147	154	162	169	177	184	191	199	206	213	221	228	235	242	250	258
6'1"	144	151	159	166	174	182	189	197	204	212	219	227	235	242	250	257	265
6'2"	148	155	163	171	179	186	194	202	210	218	225	233	241	249	256	264	272
6'3"	152	160	168	176	184	192	200	208	216	224	232	240	248	256	264	272	279

BMI CATEGORIES

- Underweight = <18.5
- Normal weight = 18.5-24.9
- Overweight = 25-29.9
- Obese = BMI of 30 or greater

Record your BMI in "Statistics: For Your Eyes Only" on page 183 in this chapter under the Current Statistics column. Your BMI number will be one gauge used to monitor your health throughout the Menopause Makeover.

CALCULATE YOUR IDEAL WEIGHT

No two bodies are alike. The combination of your body type, frame size and body composition will determine your ideal weight.

Go back to the BMI Chart and look at the weights for your height in the "normal" category (18.5 to 24.9). This will give you a healthy range to strive for.

EXAMPLE: 5'6" woman would have a normal weight range within 110 and 155 pounds.

EXAMPLE: 5'7" woman would have a normal weight range between 115 to 160 pounds

What is your healthy weight range, according to the BMI Chart?	_____to_____
What has been your healthiest weight in the past 25 years?	_____
What is your goal ideal weight for The Menopause Makeover?	_____

Record ideal weight under the Current Statistics column on page 183

UNDERSTANDING YOUR HEALTH RISKS WILL HELP YOU SET GOALS AND TRACK RESULTS.

CALCULATE YOUR WAIST-TO-HIP RATIO

To determine whether you have a healthy waist-to-hip ratio, use a fabric measuring tape and measure the circumference of your hips at the widest part of your buttocks. Then measure your waist at the smallest circumference of your natural waist, usually just above the belly button.

To determine the ratio, divide your waist measurement by your hip measurement:
_____(waist) divided by _____ (hip) = _____ waist-to-hip ratio

WAIST-TO-HIP RATIO CHART

Measurement	Health Risk
0.80 or below	Low
0.81-0.85	Moderate
0.85+	High

*What is your hip ratio?*_____

Record your hip-to-waist ratio on page 183.

*What is your health risk, if any?*_____

CALCULATE YOUR BODY FAT AND LEAN BODY MASS

Using the BMI Chart gives you a healthy weight estimate based on height and weight. Next, we will calculate how many pounds of body fat, and how many pounds of lean body mass (muscles, organs, bones) you are carrying, as well as your body fat percentage. These are excellent measurements to use to set goals for your Menopause Makeover.

To calculate lean body mass, body fat weight and body fat percentage we must first collect some numbers.

1. Total body weight _154_ x 0.732 = _12,728_ + 8.987 = _121,715_

2. Take your wrist measurement at the fullest point = _7_ divide by 3.140 = _2,229_

3. Waist measurement at your belly button = _36_ x 0.157 = _5,652_

4. Hip measurement at the fullest point = _44_ x 0.249 = _10,956_

5. Forearm measurement at the fullest point = _9,5_ x 0.434 = _4,123_

Once you calculate #1 through #5 use these numbers for the next three formulas.

Lean Body Mass Formula using calculation numbers #1 - #5

#1 121.71 + #2 2.22 - #3 5.65 - #4 10.95 + #5 4.12 = 144.65

144.65 your lean body mass in pounds

Body Fat Weight Formula using calculation numbers #1- #5

Total body weight 153 - Lean Body Mass 144 =

9 your body fat in pounds

Body Fat Percentage

Body fat weight 9 x 100 = 900 divided by your total bodyweight 154

= 5.84 your body fat percentage

How many pounds of lean body mass are you carrying? 144.65

How many pounds of fat are you carrying? 9

What is your body fat percentage? 5.84

Go to page 183 and record your lean body mass in pounds, body fat in pounds, body fat percentage under the Current Statistics column.

Having your body fat calculated underwater by a professional will give the most accurate measurement. This formula, however, is very dependable and can be used for your Menopause Makeover.

Part of the Menopause Makeover exercise commitment is to turn that fat into muscle. This will increase your metabolism, and decrease your risk of health concerns. As you start to tone up and feel better about your body, you will also get stronger – to "kick some butt" in other areas of your life.

CALCULATE YOUR CALORIE NEEDS AND SET CALORIE GOALS

This next portion is dedicated to counting calories – how many you currently consume, and what you need to consume in order to achieve your perfect weight. If you honor these numbers, you will see results. The numbers don't lie!

First, calculate your basal metabolic rate (BMR), the energy you are currently expending during physical activity, and the thermic effect of food to determine how many calories you need to maintain your current weight.

ACTUAL CALORIES YOU BURN
Calculate how many calories your body needs to maintain its current weight.

BMR + Energy Expended + Thermic Effect of Food =

Current Calories Your Body Burns Today

STEP #1 – BASAL METABOLIC RATE

Your current weight _154_ x 10 = _1540_

Take that number _1540_ + your current weight _154_ = _1694_ BMR

EXAMPLE: Current weight is 144.

144 x 10 = 1440 + 144 = 1584 (BMR)

STEP #2 – ENERGY EXPENDED DURING PHYSICAL ACTIVITY

What is your daily energy expended during physical activity?

__809__ = energy expended

(refer to the Calories Burned Per Hour chart on page 70).

1246
317
246
809

EXAMPLE:
144-pound woman does 30 minutes on the elliptical machine = 250 calories. Later that day, cleans house for 30 minutes = 150 calories. Total energy expended = 400.

STEP #3 – THERMIC EFFECT OF FOOD

Thermic effect of food (TEF) is determined by multiplying your total calorie consumption per day by 10 percent.

Total calories consumed (see Calculating Calories) _____ x 10% = _____ TEF

EXAMPLE: If I consume 2000 calories per day x 0.10 = 200 calories expended for TEF.

CALCULATING CALORIES

An easy way to figure out how many calories you consume per day is to keep a food diary for seven days counting every calorie. On the seventh day add up all your daily calorie totals and divide by seven days, giving you an average daily calorie consumption number. This strategy will give you a good average of how many total calories you are consuming daily.

STEP #4: TAKE THE PREVIOUS THREE CALCULATIONS AND APPLY

BMR _____ + Energy Expended _____ + TEF _____ =

_____ total calories used by the body to maintain your current weight.

EXAMPLE: 1584 + 400 + 200 = 2184 calories required to maintain 144 pounds.

How many calories is your body currently burning to maintain its current weight?

_____

Record this number on page 183 under the Current Statistics column.

HOW MANY CALORIES DO YOU NEED TO CONSUME TO LOSE WEIGHT?
To lose one pound, you need to lose 3,500 calories.

If you want to lose:

- ½ pound per week, subtract 250 food calories per day.
- 1 pound per week, subtract 500 food calories per day.
- 1½ pounds per week, subtract 750 food calories per day.
- 2 pounds per week, subtract 1000 food calories per day.
- Taking exercise into account: ½ pound per week, eat 125 fewer calories and move 125 calories (leisurely 30-minute walk).
- 1 pound per week, eat 250 fewer calories, move 250 more (brisk 30-minute walk).
- 1½ pounds per week, eat 375 fewer calories, move 375 calories more.
- 2 pounds per week, 500 fewer calories of food per day, 500 calories more activity (take a brisk walk and vacuum the house like a mad woman).

CALCULATE YOUR CALORIE GOAL

There are two numbers you need in order to figure out your calorie goals. First you need to calculate how many calories you need to *cut* from your diet in order to lose weight. Using this number, you can figure out how many calories you should eat every day.

HOW MANY CALORIES SHOULD YOU CUT?

First, how many pounds per week do you want to lose? _____Multiply this number by 3,500 to get the number of calories you'd need to cut in one week to achieve this goal. To determine how many calories a day you'd need to cut in order to make this happen, divide the total calories by seven.

Losing one to two pounds per week is a healthy goal. If you have more than ten to fifteen pounds to lose, you may lose more than two pounds the first few weeks. Be realistic when setting your weight loss goals. If you have 60 pounds to lose, plan on losing two pounds per week. That would take 30 weeks to meet your goal. The good news is you can use your 12-week Menopause Makeover Plan over and over until you achieve your goals.

EXAMPLE:

I want to lose 1 pound per week; that equals 3500 fewer
calories per week, or 500 calories less per day.

HOW MANY CALORIES SHOULD YOU EAT PER DAY?

Now all you have to do is subtract the number of calories you should cut from the total number of calories you need per day to maintain your weight. Keep in mind that you should never consume fewer than 1,200 calories a day, or you risk putting your body into survival mode and *holding on* to calories instead of losing them!

EXAMPLE 1:

I consume 2184 calories per day and want to lose 1 pound per week.

2184 calories – 500 calories = 1684 calories per day to lose one pound per week.

EXAMPLE 2:

I consume 2184 calories per day and want to lose 2 pounds per week.

2184 calories – 1000 calories = 1184.

It is unhealthy to consume fewer than 1200 calories per day.
My adjusted goal would be 1200 calories per day to lose up to two pounds per week.

I decide to be less aggressive and lose one pound per week. My plan is to cut 250 calories a day through exercise and eat 250 calories less to cut a total of 500 calories a day. That is a plan I can live with. When you create your plan, keep in mind your lifestyle and set reasonable goals for yourself. (You can find these calculations online at www.menopausemakeover.com)

Record your calorie cutting goals on page 183 under the 12-Week Goal column.

VISUALIZE THE NEW YOU.

VISUALIZE THE POSSIBILITIES

After you collect current information and set goals, the next step is to visualize your possibilities. If you have to lose 50 pounds to be healthy, set goals you can live with. Try losing ONE pound per week. Next year at this time, you will be at that healthy weight. It probably took years to gain that weight. Give yourself realistic goals.

I gained 25 pounds in a very short period of time. I set an aggressive goal, two pounds per week. In 12 weeks I actually lost 25 pounds. I have managed to keep off 20 pounds of that consistently, and fluctuate 5 pounds depending on holidays and travel. This is normal. I continue to practice my new healthy lifestyle by exercising 5-6 days per week and eating within my healthy calorie intake. If I find myself gaining again, I go back on the plan to keep my weight under control.

I always feel better knowing that my health is above average. It is all a balancing act. The numbers don't lie! I am still shocked to look back at my previous numbers. It feels great to have accomplished my goals. Numbers held the key to my future–and they do for you, too.

NOW THAT YOU KNOW YOUR NUMBERS, USE THEM AND BELIEVE WITH ALL YOUR HEART THAT YOU DESERVE TO BE HEALTHY.

STATISTICS: FOR YOUR EYES ONLY

Pull out that measuring tape, it is time to record your statistics. This may be the most depressing section of the Makeover. It was for me. Once I started my Menopause Makeover, these statistics were scary yet liberating. Do not share this section with anyone. It is for your eyes only.

Why do we have to torture ourselves with this horrifying exercise? Because measuring yourself – seeing it in writing – may just be the kick in the pants you need to allow you to move forward.

For years, I thought my butt was the same size it was a decade ago. *Wrong.* It was four inches bigger. My waistline had grown *six* inches thicker! After a well-needed sob session, sitting naked in the bathroom with the tape measure, I got inspired. I took that photograph of myself taken a few years earlier, when I felt and looked good, and taped it to my bathroom mirror. I made copies of the photo and carried one around in my daily planner. I also taped a copy in my Menopause Makeover Planner. I looked at the photo every day. Twelve weeks later, I once again looked like the happy girl in that picture. Once you go through menopause, that waistline needs some extra attention. After the 12-Week Plan, I got my waistline back, and my health. It was a good pinch thicker than the old days, but at least it was an hourglass again…not a basketball.

MAKEOVER TIPS:	• Be honest when calculating "your numbers."
	• Use these calculations to track your performance.
	• If you need help measuring yourself, ask a friend or loved one.

DOCUMENT YOUR STATISTICS

Drag yourself into the bathroom. Strip down. Pull out that tape measure and start recording the hard truth, *your current statistics*, on page 183. Next, set realistic goals under the "12-Week Goal" column. After your *Menopause Makeover,* come back to this page and record your results.

In just twelve weeks you can be on your way to a healthier you! These statistics will help you stay motivated, and allow you to track your goals. Find a photograph of a healthy you, after the age of 25 years old, to use as inspiration. Tape your inspiration photo on page 184.

MAKEOVER TIPS:

* Use a soft, fabric tape measure. It can be easier to have someone help you take your measurements while standing.

* Make sure your scale is on level ground. Stand on the scale first thing in the morning, naked if possible. Good calibration is important.

* Measure your bust wearing a bra, if you normally wear one.

* Measure your abdomen just under your belly button.

* Measure your calf at the maximum circumference.

* Measure your thigh at the crotch level below the fold of your buns.

* Use the BMI Chart to determine your correct body mass index.

* Wear the same clothes, or your birthday suit, when you measure again 12 weeks later.

* Pull the tape measure tight enough to stay in position, but not too tight.

* If you have blood pressure concerns, buy a blood pressure "cuff" to monitor your blood pressure. These can be purchased at most pharmacies.

* If you have cholesterol concerns, record your levels. Your doctor can give you these numbers from a blood test.

* Set realistic goals. Measurable results usually take four or more weeks.

* Take a previous photograph of yourself and tape it on page 184, "Inspirational Me." Then record the date. Twelve weeks later, place your current photograph on the same page under, "New Me."

STATISTICS: FOR YOUR EYES ONLY

Start Date _____   End Date _____

	Current	12-Week Goal	Results
Height			
Neck			
Upper arms			
Bust	40		
Waist	36		
Abdomen	42"		
Hips	46		
Waist-to-Hip Ratio			
Thighs	24		
BMI	25.		
Lean body mass	144.65		
Body fat (lbs.)	9		
Body fat (%)	5.84		
Calves			
Calories to maintain / Calories to lose			
Blood Pressure			
Cholesterol	268	↓ 200	
Weight / Ideal Weight	154 / 140		

Triglycerides   215   ↓150
LDL   171   ↓130

MAKEOVER TAKE ACTION LIST

* Do all the calculations in this chapter.
* Record these numbers.

IN YOUR ESSENTIAL PLANNER

* Use your new calorie intake goal in the 12-Week Plan.
* Subtract exercise and activity calories from food intake calories to record your total daily calorie intake in the 12-Week Plan.
* Track your results using Your Weekly Progress Report.

NOW THAT YOU SEE THE NUMBERS, VISUALIZE, VISUALIZE, VISUALIZE! IF YOU THINK ABOUT YOUR GOALS, YOU CAN ACHIEVE THEM!

| Chapter 12 | # Setting Goals
If You Write It Down,
You Can Make It Happen |

After reading Part One, you are armed with knowledge. After doing the personal calculations, you are empowered with truth. Knowledge combined with truth is a winning formula for setting goals.

SET GOALS FOR YOUR 12-WEEK MAKEOVER

Setting goals will allow you to track successes and challenges. This is your personalized portion of the Menopause Makeover.

For some unexplained reason, I have set annual goals since I was 12 years old. In those early years, my goals were simple: get straight A's on my report card; practice the piano; learn how to sew so I could make a pair of hot pants (my mom would not let me buy them); keep out of trouble; protect my brother and his hamster; play Liddle Kiddles with my friends. I witnessed at any early age that if I made a list of goals inspired by my dreams, they almost always miraculously happened. Goal-setting works, no matter what your age.

Now my goals are larger, encompassing more areas of my life. Every year on New Year's Day, I sit down and write goals. I include long- and short-term goals. I have personal goals, and goals for my relationship. Each year I save these goals. I love to look back and see the power of realized goals. My life is richer in all areas, thanks to goal-setting.

The process of asking what you want or need to be happy is a powerful exercise. This is often difficult for women. We are committed to others – often forgetting, or not even knowing, what we need to make us happy. Goal-setting can change your life, whether you need to manage menopause symptoms, revamp your image, create or recreate a stimulating career, or work on a more intimate relationship.

In earlier chapters you were asked to fill out portions of this section, so you have already started. Take some quiet time and reflect on your goals. Be honest, dig deep, and dream big!

MAKEOVER TIPS	❋ Identify what you want. ❋ Write it down. ❋ Be committed to taking the action needed to make it possible. ❋ Believe in yourself. ❋ Believe your goals are possible. ❋ Tap into your dreams. ❋ When you have quiet time, visualize your goals happening. What will your life look like? How will you feel? ❋ Be grateful for goals realized. ❋ Be grateful for lessons learned from unrealized goals. ❋ Be excited about your life embracing these new goals; this energy creates results. ❋ Be an inspiration to yourself and others.
MAKEOVER TAKE ACTION LIST	❋ Review your goals weekly. ❋ Add new goals. ❋ Share your goals with others – being accountable to others can yield faster results.
IN YOUR ESSENTIAL PLANNER	❋ Record all actions to achieve your goals in your Month-at-a-Glance Planner. ❋ Write about your goals in your Journal.

IF YOU WRITE IT DOWN, YOU CAN MAKE IT HAPPEN!

YOUR PERSONAL GOALS

Start date: _____ End date: _____

Overall Menopause Makeover Goal

What is your ACTION plan to achieve this goal?

Hormones

How will you address menopause symptoms?

What health concerns need attention?

What action will you take to manage these health concerns?

Nutrition

What are your nutrition goals?

How will you achieve these goals?

What are your big "food challenges"?

How will you conquer these challenges?

What supplements have you chosen for the 12-Week Plan?

What is your daily calorie intake to achieve or maintain a healthy weight?

How will you achieve this?

Exercise

What daily exercise activities have you chosen for the 12-week plan?

How long will you do these exercises each day?

How many days per week?

What is your target heart rate?

What was your health rating result from the "One Mile Walking Test"?

How will you improve this rating?

If you dread exercising, how will you overcome this attitude?

Beauty

What are your overall beauty goals?

How will you achieve them?

What are your goals for:
Skincare regime

Hairstyle/color

Your Wardrobe

What age-embracing tips will you practice (refer to page 86)?

What makeup tips will you incorporate (refer to page 99)?

What styling tips will you incorporate (refer to page 103)?

Emotions

What areas of your emotional life need a Makeover?

How will you address:
Crankiness

Moodiness

Depression

Memory loss/fuzzy thinking

Stress

Relationships

What is the most important goal regarding your primary love relationship?

What relationships need extra attention?
Family

Friends

Co-workers

Neighbors

Others

How will you address these relationship challenges?

Spirituality & Happiness

How will you nurture your spirit?

How will you nurture your passions, and purpose in life?

How will you make a difference in your life?

How will you create happiness in your life?

Review all areas of happiness (page 150)
What are your short-term happiness goals?

What are your long-term happiness goals?

What dreams do you want to manifest in your lifetime?

How can you achieve them?

How can you simplify your life?

In which areas of your life do you need to practice forgiveness?

When you successfully complete *The Menopause Makeover,* how will you reward yourself?

Living Your Dreams

List your dreams:

How can you start making these dreams realities?

From the Happiness Questionnaire, what areas can you improve?

What is your action plan?

Action Plan
Areas that needs to be addressed:
Health

Love (with someone special)

Spirituality

Self-esteem

Work

Money (Do you feel safe?)

Hobbies

Friends

Relatives

Children

Home

Travel/adventure

Education/learning

Neighborhood

Giving

Creativity

Each week review this list and start incorporating an "action" to create improvement. Set short-term goals (1 month, 3 months and 6 months):

Set long-term goals (1 year and 5 years):

Refer to your list daily. Visualize goals happening. Update your goals. When a new desire comes up, add it to the list. Create positive goals. Prioritize your goals. Have small and large goals. Some will happen faster than others. Some may be complex and need time. Set realistic goals.

Every day, record in your Essential Planner the actions needed to achieve your goals.

TAKING THE VOW: SAYING "I DO" TO THE NEW YOU

The Menopause Makeover embraces celebration! You have taken the steps to personalize your Menopause Makeover, and set goals. It is time to say "I do" to the new you! Just like marriage, taking a vow (a solemn promise to perform a certain act) can be a fun process to verbalize your Menopause Makeover commitment to yourself and the people you love. Giving yourself a party launching your Menopause Makeover is a wonderful way to celebrate your commitment to the journey you are about to begin. Selecting an attractive reward for accomplishing your goals is a great incentive to stay on-course.

Your Menopause Makeover can take as much effort as planning a wedding. Why not incorporate some of the fun stuff weddings include? Planning a party with your close friends and family is a fantastic way to show the world you are serious about your Menopause Makeover commitment. Perhaps your friends are struggling with menopause as well? Invite them to join you in the Menopause Makeover—you can all celebrate the start of your journey together!

CELEBRATE THE NEW YOU

Personalize your Menopause Makeover using a party theme unique to you. Are you an earthy-type person? If so, plan an "Overnight Backyard Camping Party" with a few good girlfriends. Are you a diva? Perhaps the "Diva Party" will be the perfect fit for you. Customize your party, and celebrate *you*. Here are few ideas to get you started:

Afternoon tea party

Invite friends to enjoy "afternoon tea" Saturday or Sunday between 3pm and 5pm.

Margarita hot-flash fiesta

Dust off the blender and whip up some yummy margaritas. Announce when you have a hot flash, and everyone has to take a sip of their margarita.

Spa party

Book manicures and pedicures at your local salon or spa. Invite your girlfriends to an afternoon of pampering dedicated to your Menopause Makeover. Or book a manicurist and pedicurist to come to your home for an evening of luxury. If you really want to go all-out, book one of the many resort spas that host spa parties for groups. Make your Menopause Makeover an event!

Makeover and a meal

This is always a crowd-pleaser. Book a makeup artist and invite your girlfriends over for dinner. As you enjoy the evening with good friends, everyone gets a personalized makeup-makeover. Take before and after photos. Often a Mary Kay or Avon representative can provide products and consultation for the group as you party.

Diva Party

Embrace your inner diva with a Diva dinner party. Everyone must dress as a diva. Hire your own paparazzi.

THE RING: YOUR COMMITMENT TO YOU

Before you take The Menopause Makeover vow, select a ring that you will wear on your right hand the next 12 weeks. I located my grandmother's wedding ring. I had it sized and polished. As I wear her ring on my right-hand ring finger, I am inspired by her memory. You may have a college ring that holds good memories. Perhaps you want to purchase a new ring for this occasion. Or maybe someone special in your life would like to give you a ring to honor your Menopause Makeover.

Next, take the Menopause Makeover vow. You can read this vow privately to yourself or in front of loved ones.

The Menopause Makeover Vow

I promise to accept responsibility for my health.

I promise to love my natural beauty.

I promise to work hard at achieving my goals.

I promise to have an open mind to what is possible.

I promise to take action toward positive change.

I promise to nourish my body with healthy food.

I promise to exercise and stay active.

I promise to seek support when I need it.

I promise to forgive those who have hurt me.

I promise to be grateful for my blessings.

I promise to celebrate my spirit every day.

I promise to encourage others.

I promise to manifest good things for myself.

I promise to live in the present moment.

I promise to love myself in sickness and in health, for richer or poorer, forevermore.

After you take the Menopause Makeover vow, slip that special ring on your right ring finger. You just made a big commitment to your health, beauty and life.

TWELVE WEEKS FROM NOW, YOU WILL LOOK AND FEEL BETTER. NO MATTER WHAT YOUR RESULTS, YOU ARE MAKING POSITIVE CHANGE TO YOUR LIFE.

THE MENOPAUSE MAKEOVER REWARD

Congratulations! You have made an important vow to change your life. Select a reward to enjoy when you complete your Menopause Makeover. It can be inexpensive, or expensive. It should be something special to you. You are about to begin 12 weeks of life-changing action. There will be struggles, challenges and frustrations – along with big successes. All of life's transitions are interwoven with ups and downs. Having a reward at the end of this journey can be a great motivator. My initial reward was fitting into the beautiful wedding gown my mother had given me for my special day! The next time I did the 12-Week Plan, my reward was a new wardrobe for my new body. My husband went shopping with me and helped pick out some flattering, sexy outfits.

Your Menopause Makeover journey will also provide rewards you cannot buy. Treat yourself when you complete the Menopause Makeover.

Now it's time to begin *your* Menopause Makeover!

MAKEOVER TIPS

* Select a party theme that is personal to you. Be proud to celebrate your new beginning. If you are happy about it, everyone will be happy for you.
* Get excited about the next 12 weeks—have fun!
* Take your vow seriously.
* Wear your ring joyfully. The Menopause Makeover is about a commitment to you.

IN YOUR ESSENTIAL PLANNER

* Tape a picture of your reward on Your Menopause Makeover Reward page.
* Schedule your Menopause Makeover party in Your Month-at-a-Glance Planner.
* Track results in Your Weekly Progress Report.

PART 3

Your Menopause Makeover Essential Planner: 12 Weeks to a New You

	The Essential Planner
Chapter 13	Charting Your Success

So now you are informed, you've done your calculations and set goals, and you made a commitment to your Menopause Makeover. This section provides the tools you need to chart your success. If you write it down, you can create it, be it, do it and achieve it.

The Menopause Makeover Tools

- **Month-at-a-Glance**: use this calendar to keep track of your appointments.

- **Your Menopause Makeover Contacts**: record contact information for your support group and makeover contacts.

- **Medical Forms**: prepare your medical forms from Chapter One for your next doctor's appointment, and review the medical tests for your age group.

- **Menopause Makeover Food Plan**: prepare your food plan every week to stay on track with your nutrition goals.

- **Menopause Makeover Shopping List:** use the shopping list to ensure that basket is loaded with healthy food.

- **Menopause Makeover Daily Meal Diary:** make a habit of using daily. It is one of the most important tools for your makeover.

- Your 12-Week Plan: document medications, hormones, and exercise daily
- Weekly Progress Report: chart your progress with this weekly report
- Your Gratitude List: record the things/people you are grateful.
- Your Menopause Makeover Reward: stay motivated with this reminder of how you'll reward yourself when you achieve your goals.
- Journal Pages: keep a journal of your feelings.
- **Notes:** if you have an idea, question, need a reminder jot it down.

All of these tools will help you stay on track for a successful makeover. While you can write in these actual pages, you may want to use them as a template to create your own Menopause Makeover binder—you can copy the Month-at-a-Glance, Food Plan, Shopping List, Daily Meal Diary, 12-Week Plan and Weekly Progress Report so that you will have enough to use for all 12 weeks of the Makeover. Or you can download these forms from my website at www.Menopause-Makeover.com.

This chapter is dedicated to making your dreams come true!

ACKNOWLEDGE YOUR SUCCESSES.

YOUR MONTH-AT-A-GLANCE PLANNER

Doctor visits, exercise dates, new beauty regimes, shopping dates, lunch with supportive friends, meetings with your spiritual group, and dates with your loved ones—there's so much to keep track of!

Use this monthly planner to keep track of all your appointments, and witness your transformation during the *12-Week Menopause Makeover!*

MONTH _____

Sunday	Monday	Tuesday	Wednesday	Thursday	Friday	Saturday

MAKEOVER TIPS

1	Record all activities and appointments for your 12-Week Menopause Makeover on the Month-at-a-Glance Planner.
2	"Starting weight" is your original weight when you start the 12-Week Plan.
3	Track your menopause symptoms. Use the chart on page 10.
4	Be honest with your emotions.
5	Set goals in the exercise section. For example, are you just trying to include exercise in your life? Or are you trying to increase intensity and duration for better results? Push yourself – you will be amazed at the outcome. If you get bored, ask a friend to join or change your activity.
6	Purchase a heart rate monitor watch, if you don't use exercise equipment with this information. Your heart rate will allow you to track and monitor intensity. This is a great tool to use when exercising and setting goals.
7	You can use the Calories Burned Per Hour chart on page 70 to calculate calories in "other activity."
8	If you wake up and eat at 6 am, make sure you have a mid-morning snack. If you eat breakfast at 8-9 a.m., do not add a mid-morning snack.
9	Calculating calories is one of the most important tasks you can do in this journal entry. After the first couple of weeks it will become easier, because you will know the calorie information for your favorite foods. Stick with it and it will pay off.
10	Be honest with yourself regarding the areas that need work. Acknowledging challenges is the first step to overcoming them.

YOUR MENOPAUSE MAKEOVER CONTACTS

Keep a list of all Menopause Makeover contacts. Include everyone from your doctor (gynecologist, eye doctor, dentist, dermatologist) to the lab, pharmacy, health food store, practitioner, hair stylist, exercise location, trainer, and your spiritual or support group.

Name	Phone Number	E-mail	Address

MENOPAUSE MAKEOVER MEDICAL FORMS

CURRENT EMOTIONAL AND PHYSICAL CONCERNS

List your current emotional and physical concerns, such as vision changes, skin issues, high blood pressure, weight gain, migraines, hair loss, mood swings, depression, fatigue, panic attacks, difficulty with sex and low libido.

1

2

3

4

5

6

7

8

9

10

YOUR PERSONAL MEDICAL HISTORY

Document YOUR medical history.
Example: Pregnancy complications, allergies, migraines, high blood pressure, endometriosis, fibroids, diabetes, broken bones, past surgeries, injuries, fatigue, seizures, asthma, infertility, incontinence, losing height, hair loss, dizziness, hospitalization, mental health problems, cancer, arthritis, history of smoking

YOUR FAMILY MEDICAL HISTORY

Genetics can affect treatment choices and offer you the opportunity to prevent future problems. Discuss your family medical history with your doctor. What diseases run in your family? Check off the appropriate.

☐ Heart disease	☐ Depression	☐ Memory loss
☐ High blood pressure	☐ Diabetes	☐ Depression
☐ Glaucoma	☐ Allergies	☐ Hair loss
☐ Blood clots	☐ Alzheimer's	☐ Obesity
☐ Stroke	☐ Arthritis	☐ Endometriosis
☐ Elevated cholesterol	☐ Challenging menopause	☐ Thyroid problems
☐ Breast cancer	☐ Chronic fatigue	☐ Autoimmune disease
☐ Uterine cancer	☐ Osteoporosis	☐ Alcoholism/Drug Abuse
☐ Ovarian cancer	☐ Migraines	☐ Incontinence
☐ List any other cancers	☐ Endocrine issues	☐ Bladder problems
☐ Fibroids	☐ Kidney problems	☐ Hysterectomy
		☐ Gallbladder disease

Other cancers:

Autoimmune disease (please specify):

List any other genetic diseases that run in your family:

CURRENT MEDICATIONS

List medications (both Prescription and Over-the-counter),
Vitamins, Minerals and Herbs You Currently Take

1

2

3

4

5

6

7

8

9

11

12

13

14

15

MENOPAUSE MAKEOVER FOOD PLAN

A food plan is a great way to stick to your Makeover! Use the
sample plan to create your own customized food plan.

SAMPLE FOOD PLAN

Based on 1,200 calories per day

Monday	Tuesday	Wednesday	Thursday	Friday	Saturday	Sunday
Breakfast						
½ cup strawberries ½ cup low-fat cottage cheese coffee	½ cup oatmeal ½ scoop protein powder ½ cup blueberries ½ cup soymilk coffee	protein shake	1 egg hardboiled 3oz lean ham coffee	½ cup fruit ½ cup cottage cheese coffee	low-fat yogurt coffee	baked frittata (see recipe)
Morning Snack						
100-calorie protein bar	½ protein shake	½ cup fruit ½ cup cottage cheese	100-calorie protein bar	½ protein shake	100-calorie protein bar	½ cup fruit ½ cup cottage cheese
Lunch						
1 cup veggie 6 oz grilled chicken breast (meat only, grilled or broiled)	4 oz tuna ½ whole wheat pita pocket light mayo ½ cup fruit	1 cup lean turkey chili 1 medium apple	crabmeat pita ½ whole wheat pita pocket 4 oz crabmeat, 1 tsp light mayo	chicken salad 6 oz grilled chicken & lettuce with veggies	1 veggie burger 1 slice of whole wheat bread	chicken curry salad (see recipe) sparkling water

Afternoon Snack						
low-fat string cheese	1 oz cashews 1 small apple	mocha shake (see recipe)	1 oz macadamia nuts	4 oz tuna, light mayo, 2 melba toasts	low-fat string cheese ½ cup fruit	2 hardboiled eggs stuffed with hummus sprinkle paprika for spice
Dinner						
6 oz pork chop 1 cup broccoli ½ cup couscous	6 oz grilled salmon 1 cup veggie baby lettuce & 1 tbsp low-fat dressing	6 oz chicken grilled 1 cup veggie ½ cup brown rice	6 oz halibut 1 cup asparagus 1 cup wild rice	6 oz pork tenderloin salad with low-fat dressing	chicken & veggie fondue (see recipe) lettuce & 1 tbsp low-fat dressing 6 oz white wine	stir-fry chicken & veggies small salad
Evening Snack						
low-fat yogurt	3.5 oz red wine low-fat string cheese	2 oz turkey lunch meat small pear	protein shake	fruit low-fat string cheese	fruit & low-fat yogurt	100-calorie protein bar
Monday	Tuesday	Wednesday	Thursday	Friday	Saturday	Sunday

MAKEOVER TIPS:

- Don't let four hours pass without eating.
- Drink water throughout the day.
- Eat protein with each meal and most snacks.
- If you "crash" (blood sugar drops from waiting too long to eat), grab one of these snacks: Fruits, low-fat string cheese, low-fat cottage cheese, sliced deli turkey, hardboiled egg stuffed with hummus, 100 calorie protein bar, 5 Nabisco Nilla Wafers, ½ cup of sorbet with ½ cup berries, 25 pistachios, 1 Yoplait light smoothie, ½ mini bagel with 1 oz. salmon, 50 Edamame (soybeans), celery and hummus dip.

FOOD PLAN

Based on _____ calories per day

Monday	Tuesday	Wednesday	Thursday	Friday	Saturday	Sunday
			Breakfast			
			Morning Snack			
			Lunch			
			Afternoon Snack			
			Dinner			
			Evening Snack			

MENOPAUSE MAKEOVER SHOPPING LIST

Once you've determined your food plan, create a shopping list to stock your fridge with everything you need to be successful with your goals. Check off the foods you need in each category.

Protein

- [ ] Fish & seafood
- [ ] White-meat poultry
- [ ] Low-fat milk
- [ ] Low-fat yogurt
- [ ] Low-fat cottage cheese
- [ ] Low-fat cheese
- [ ] Eggs
- [ ] Egg whites
- [ ] Beans
- [ ] Pork tenderloin
- [ ] Soy
- [ ] Lean Beef
- [ ] Protein shake
- [ ] Protein bar

Other

Fats

- [ ] Nuts (almonds, walnuts, pecans, cashews)
- [ ] Peanuts
- [ ] Fish (salmon, halibut, flounder, crab, tuna, trout)
- [ ] Avocado
- [ ] Olives
- [ ] Olive oil
- [ ] Safflower oil
- [ ] Flaxseed Oil

Other

FEED THE HEALTHY YOU.

Carbohydrates

- ☐ Bran cereal
- ☐ Oatmeal
- ☐ Oat bran
- ☐ All-bran
- ☐ Shredded wheat cereal
- ☐ Legumes (kidney beans, lentils, pinto beans, chickpeas)
- ☐ Fruit (apples, plums, oranges, raisins)

- ☐ Veggies (broccoli, yams, sweet potato)
- ☐ Plain yogurt
- ☐ Skim milk
- ☐ Soy beverage
- ☐ Brown rice
- ☐ Basmati rice
- ☐ Couscous
- ☐ Rice cakes

- ☐ Whole-grain breads
- ☐ Whole-grain pasta
- ☐ Rye bread
- ☐ Fruit juices without added sugar

Other

High-Fiber Foods

- ☐ Celery
- ☐ Apples
- ☐ Strawberries
- ☐ Blueberries
- ☐ Pears
- ☐ Beans
- ☐ Lentils
- ☐ Oatmeal
- ☐ Oat bran

- ☐ Nuts
- ☐ Rice bran
- ☐ Peas
- ☐ Carrots
- ☐ Cucumbers
- ☐ Celery
- ☐ Tomatoes
- ☐ Zucchini
- ☐ Whole wheat breads
- ☐ Brown rice

- ☐ Barley
- ☐ Couscous
- ☐ Rye
- ☐ Cabbage
- ☐ Brussels sprouts
- ☐ Cauliflower
- ☐ Beets

Other

Beverages

☐ Water   ☐ Juice (no sugar added)   ☐ Red wine

☐ Coffee

Other

Supplements

☐ Calcium/vitamin D   ☐ Multi-vitamin   ☐ Omega-3

Other

Low-Calorie Snacks

☐ 100-calorie cookies   ☐ 100-calorie Popsicle*

Other

ALWAYS CARRY HEALTHY SNACKS ON THE ROAD.

Protein-Rich Snacks

☐ Advantage protein shakes ☐ Protein bars ☐ Protein powder

Other

✧✧✧

DRINK AN EXTRA GLASS OF WATER TODAY.

✧✧✧

MENOPAUSE MAKEOVER DAILY MEAL PLAN

Goal: 40% protein; 35% Carbs; 25% Fats per serving	Calorie	Protein	Carbs	Fat	Fiber
Breakfast					
Time: _____ (Eat within one hour of waking) List foods below					
Lunch					
Time: _____ List foods below					
Afternoon Snack					
Time: _____ List foods below					
Dinner					
Time: _____ List foods below					
Evening Snack					
Time: _____ List foods below					
Totals for the day					

Food Servings

Food	Servings Per Day	Portion Size
Protein	5-6	Size of your palm
Carbs	3-5	slice or 1.2 cup
Fruits	2-5	med., ½ cup chopped, ½ cup juice
Vegetables	3-5	1 cup raw or ½ cup cooked
Fats	5-6	Size of your thumb
Dairy	2, nonfat	½ cup
Protein Snacks	1-2 per day	(power bar, power shake, protein powder)
Water	6-8	8 fluid ounces
Coffee	Less than 2	1 cup
Alcohol	Less than 6 ounces	

Daily Calories Consumed

Food Calories – Exercise Calories – Activity Calories = Daily Calories Consumed

YOUR 12-WEEK PLAN

Week

| 1 | 2 | 3 | 4 | 5 | 6 | 7 | 8 | 9 | 10 | 11 | 12 |

Date   Day of Week

Starting Weight   Current Weight   Goal Weight

Hormones (record daily)

Estrogen	AM	PM	Progesterone	AM	PM

Monthly Cycle   ☐ Yes ☐ No

Current Medications

What menopause symptoms are you experiencing?

How do you feel emotionally today?

Exercise

Cardio: Goal, 20-30 minutes a day, 5-6 days a week.   **Strength building**: Goal, 2-3 times per week or daily.

Cardio	Strength building
Weekly goal	Weekly goal
What type of exercise:	What type of exercise:
Intensity: ☐ Low ☐ Medium ☐ High	Intensity: ☐ Low ☐ Medium ☐ High
For how long:	For how long:
Heart rate average:	Heart rate average:
Did I succeed? ☐ Yes ☐ No	Did I succeed? ☐ Yes ☐ No
Calories burned: Time of day:	Calories burned: Time of day:
	Other Activity: Calories Burned

YOUR WEEKLY PROGRESS

Date

Day of Week

Starting Weight

Current Weight

Goal Weight

Weight difference from last week

If your weight is less than last week, to what do you attribute this success? Cutting portions? Counting calories? Cutting out junk food? More exercise? Symptom treatment?

If your weight is more than last week, why?

What was the most difficult part of your makeover last week?

How are your menopausal symptoms: ☐ the same   ☐ better   ☐ worse
How are you addressing your symptoms?

What do you enjoy most about your exercise routine?

What do you not like about your exercise routine?

What can you do to make your exercise program more successful or enjoyable?

Have you noticed a pattern in your eating habits that you need to change? ☐ Yes ☐ No
What do you need to change in your meal planning to meet your goals?

Where do you excel with your meal planning?

Where do you fail with your meal planning?

What are your exercise and eating goals for the upcoming week?

Overall, how would you rate your emotional health this past week?

What beauty goals did you accomplish this week?

SEE THE FINISH LINE AT ALL TIMES. MOVE FORWARD KNOWING YOUR END RESULTS.

YOUR GRATITUDE LIST

List everything for which you are grateful.
Continue to add throughout your Menopause Makeover.

THIS IS YOUR CHANCE TO LIVE YOUR DREAMS.

YOUR MENOPAUSE MAKEOVER REWARD

Tape a 4x6 photograph of your Menopause Makeover reward here.

JOURNAL PAGES

NOTES

| Chapter 14 | Menopause Makeover Recipes and Menus |

One of the biggest adjustments you need to make to be successful with your menopause makeover is creating new eating habits. What foods you eat can make the difference between a smooth menopause transition and a bumpy road. The Menopause Makeover Food Pyramid allows you the flexibility to eat delicious foods while improving your health and helping you lose weight. I have included a few of my favorite recipes to demonstrate how eating according to the food pyramid can still be incredibly satisfying and delicious. There is also room to add your own favorite Makeover recipes that honor the food pyramid. Have fun with food! Be creative, and bon appetite.

FAVORITE MAKEOVER BREAKFASTS

BAKED BREAKFAST FRITTATA

The level of protein and fiber will keep you feeling full for hours. This meal honors The Menopause Makeover Food Pyramid--it is perfectly balanced, low in calories and the perfect way to start the day.

6-8 servings
Prep time = 30 minutes

1 tablespoon olive oil
1-1/2 cups potatoes cut in 1/2-inch cubes
1-1/2 cups chopped cooked LEAN ham (8 oz.)
3/4-cup (3 oz.) low-fat shredded cheddar cheese
8 eggs slightly beaten (or two 8-oz. cartons of egg product)
1/3 cup low-fat milk
Chili peppers
2 teaspoons fresh oregano

1/4 teaspoon salt
4-oz. can diced green onions
2 teaspoons of psyllium husks (you can buy this powdered fiber – it has no taste – at a health food store or grocery store like Whole Foods)
1/2 of a 7-oz. jar of roasted red sweet peppers cut into thin strips
1-1/2 cups salsa
1/4 cup fresh cilantro
3 sprigs of parsley

Directions

* Preheat oven: 350 degrees.
* In a 10-inch oven-safe skillet, cook the potatoes in hot olive oil, uncovered over medium heat for 5 minutes. Stir occasionally. Then cover and cook for another 5 minutes until tender.
* Remove from heat and mix in the ham and 1/2 cup of cheddar cheese.
* In a mixing bowl, stir together the eggs, milk, chili peppers, oregano, salt, onions and psyllium husks. Then pour into the skillet and mix together. Lay the pepper strips on top of the frittata.
* Bake uncovered for 25-30 minutes.
* Sprinkle the top with 1/4 cup of cheddar cheese. In a separate pan, stir salsa and cilantro together and heat.
* Cut the frittata into wedges, place the parsley as decoration next to the wedge and serve with the salsa mixture. Serve on a smaller dish with a lovely wine glass filled with chilled water and a twist of lemon.

Calories 196 / Protein 17 grams / Carbs 11 grams / Fat 8 grams / Fiber 2 grams

COFFEE MOCHA PROTEIN SHAKE

1 cup soy milk or skim milk
2 scoops of whey chocolate protein powder
2 teaspoons instant coffee, or a shot of espresso
1 teaspoon of vanilla extract
1 cup ice cubes

Directions

* In a blender, combine all ingredients and blend until smooth. Enjoy!

Using soy milk: Calories 243 / Protein 29.2 grams / Carbs 15.9 grams / Fat 6.6 grams / Fiber 4.2 grams
Using skim milk: Calories 206 / Protein 28.3 grams / Carbs 16.7 grams / Fat 1.7 grams / Fiber 1 gram

MAKEOVER TIPS:

You can pre-make this shake and refrigerate, then pour into an insulated thermos, so it will be ready to enjoy mid-afternoon.

FAVORITE MAKEOVER LUNCHES

Once you add the lettuce, pita or wrap this meal honors The Menopause Makeover Food Pyramid food ratios of 35% protein, 40% carbohydrates, and 25% fats. This yummy recipe helps you fight the menopause midsection and love handles!

By using curry, this scrumptious recipe contains enhanced health benefits. Curry is a blend of various spices, with the most common mixture being turmeric, ground cumin, cardamom and coriander. Curry boasts anti-inflammatory properties and can help promote neurological health.

With the addition of other healthy ingredients such as onions, apples and chicken (an excellent lean meat choice), this salad is a healthy yet delicious way to jumpstart your summer.

I like to serve this salad with sliced, chilled pears or apples on the side, and sparkling water with a sprig of mint ... yummy!

CHICKEN CURRY SALAD

6 servings
prep time = 20 minutes, allow time to chill before serving

1/2 cup low-fat cottage cheese	2 cups cooked chicken, breast
1 teaspoon curry powder	meat only, chopped
2 spring onions, large	Dash of pepper
1/4 cup walnut halves, chopped	¼ cup scallions, thinly sliced
1 small apple, peeled and cubed	

Directions

* Puree the cottage cheese in a food processor. Add curry powder and pepper. Mix well. Puree to the desired consistency. I prefer a thicker puree, so be careful not to over-process this mixture.

* Add onions, walnut halves, apples and chopped chicken to the curry mixture.

* Serve on a bed of baby lettuce, or in 1/2 whole-wheat pita, or 1/2 a whole-wheat wrap.

* Serve chilled. Please note, it is best to make this recipe a few hours before serving. Sprinkle thinly sliced scallions on top.

Calories 193 (without the pita or wrap) / Protein 26.3 grams / Carbs 6.3 grams
Fat 7.2 grams / Fiber 1.5 grams

This is my all-time favorite chili recipe. The good news is that chili is not only comfort food, but it can be healthy, too! Chili contains lots of protein. (This recipe is made with turkey, so it is a leaner alternative to ground beef.) And chili can help you lose weight. The "capsaicin," a colorless compound found in the chilies used to season this dish, can increase your metabolic rate by increasing your body heat production. Chili is also high in iron thanks to the turkey and beans and has vitamin C thanks to the tomatoes, peppers and chilies. Plus, it's a great source of fiber that helps keep you full for a long time after eating. Enjoy the healthy benefits of chili!

TURKEY CHILI

8-10 servings
Prep time = 30 minutes

2 medium onions, chopped (1 cup)
1 tablespoon vegetable oil
2 tablespoons chopped fresh garlic
1 medium red bell pepper, chopped (1 cup)
1 medium green bell pepper, chopped (1 cup)
2 pounds ground turkey
2 tablespoons ground cumin
1 tablespoon dried oregano leaves
1 tablespoon chili powder
1 can (4 ounces) chopped
green chilies, drained

2 jalapeño chilies, seeded and chopped
28-oz. can of whole Roma (plum) tomatoes
3 cups water for thick meaty chili,
or 4 cups for "soupier" chili
2 cans (15 ounces) black beans, drained
1 can (15 to 16 ounces) kidney beans, drained
Salt and pepper to taste
Sweet onions, sliced
Low-fat sour cream

Directions

- Cook the onions in vegetable oil in a large saucepan over medium heat for about 10 minutes or until the onions are tender.
- Add garlic and the green and red bell peppers, cook 2 to 3 minutes.
- Add turkey and cook 3 to 4 minutes or until the turkey is no longer pink.
- Add cumin, oregano, chili powder, green chilies, jalapeño chilies, tomatoes and water. Reduce heat to low.
- Cover and simmer about 30 minutes.
- Add beans; simmer 15 to 20 minutes longer. I simmer for a total of 2 hours for a rich flavor.
- To serve, add sliced sweet onions to the top and a dab of low-fat sour cream.

If you want to make this recipe spicy, add one whole red habeñero or one whole serrano chili (deveined, deseeded and chopped). Or if you like a Tex-Mex flavor, add an envelope of taco seasoning as you simmer this recipe.

Calories 175 / Protein 15 grams / Carbs 13 grams / Fat 6 grams / Fiber 5 grams

FAVORITE MAKEOVER DINNERS

ROMANTIC DINNER FOR TWO

This is a fun romantic meal—it not only helps with step two of your Makeover, but will help rekindle the romance for step six, too!

The menu

- Tempting beginning: Chilled grapes and fruit.
- Wine: Red (Zinfandel).
- Main course: Chicken and veggie fondue with dipping sauces.
- Sinful endings: Strawberries dipped in dark chocolate.

CHICKEN AND VEGGIE FONDUE WITH DIPPING SAUCES

This dinner is low in fat and high in protein.

2 servings   Prep time = 15 minutes

1 pound skinless and boneless chicken breasts 2 cups cauliflower	2 cups broccoli dipping sauces

Directions

- Cut the chicken breasts and vegetables into bite-sized portions.
- Place the chicken in a serving dish separate from the vegetables. Refrigerate until ready to serve.
- Place your favorite dipping sauces in separate serving dishes.
- If you are serving this meal in a hotel room with a kitchenette, bring the chilled food in a cooler.

Suggested dipping sauces

Peppercorn, honey-mustard, peanut satay, sesame garlic, BBQ and/or teriyaki sauce.
Purchase these sauces pre-made and keep your special evening simple.

Fondue preparation

- Half fill the fondue pot with vegetable oil.
- Then pour the measured oil into a saucepan on the stovetop and heat the oil to 375 degrees F. You will know the oil is ready when you drop a piece of bread in and it browns in 30 seconds.
- Pour the oil back into the fondue pot and light the burner.
- Place the chicken, vegetables and dipping sauces around the fondue pot.
- Start cooking your dinner. Each piece of chicken should cook in the fondue pot 1-2 minutes.

DARK CHOCOLATE DIPPED STRAWBERRIES

4 servings
Prep time = 15 minutes

4 ounces semi-sweet chocolate
1 small carton of medium-sized whole strawberries

Directions

* Microwave chocolate in a glass bowl, stopping after 30 seconds, then every 10 seconds until almost melted.
* Stir until smooth and glossy.
* Wash strawberries and pat them dry (any moisture from the fruit will spoil the texture of the melted chocolate).
* Dip each strawberry into the melted chocolate, covering the lower half of the strawberry.
* Place on a baking sheet lined with wax paper.
* Refrigerate for at least 1 hour.

Per chocolate strawberry - Calories 48 / Protein 0.5 grams / Carbs 6.8 grams
Fat 18 grams / Fiber 1.1 grams /

After you have enjoyed cooking your fondue dinner, bring out the dark chocolate or chocolate-dipped strawberries for a sinful ending. Healthy dark chocolate has a cocoa content of 60-70 percent or higher. Eating 2 ounces (50 grams) a day of plain chocolate with a minimum content of 60 percent chocolate solids, can be beneficial to health – providing protection against heart disease, high blood pressure, and many other health hazards – as well as providing vitamins, and essential trace elements and nutrients such as iron, calcium and potassium. A 1-1/2-ounce square of chocolate may have as many cancer-fighting antioxidants as a 5-ounce glass of red wine. And chocolate stimulates the secretion of endorphins, producing a pleasurable sensation. So don't feel guilty, enjoy some dark chocolate!

TIPS FOR SELECTING YOUR WINE

* The wine should not be sweeter than the chocolate you are serving.
* When pairing wines with chocolate, the stronger the chocolate, the more full-bodied the wine should be. For example, a bittersweet chocolate tends to pair well with an intense Zinfandel.
* Don't forget to play your favorite music, light plenty of candles, and mist yourself with sensual perfume.

ROASTED TURKEY

This recipe is perfect for entertaining, or makes a great dinner for two with healthy leftovers.
10-12 servings

12-14 pound whole turkey, giblets removed
A couple sprigs each of fresh thyme,
oregano, sage and parsley
3 tablespoons olive oil
2 tablespoons dry white wine

2 tablespoons paprika
Fresh ground pepper to taste
3 small oranges, unpeeled and cut into wedges
2 onions, cut into wedges
1 cup of low-fat, low-sodium chicken broth

Directions

- Preheat the oven to 325 degrees F.
- Lift up the skin covering the turkey breast.
- Slip the thyme, oregano, sage and parsley underneath the skin.
- Combine the oil, wine, paprika and pepper. Rub this mixture over the surface of the turkey.
- Place the oranges and onions inside the turkey.
- Place turkey, breast side down, in a roasting pan. Pour chicken broth into the bottom of the pan. Cover loosely with aluminum foil.
- Roast for 20-25 minutes per pound, basting periodically.
- Halfway through cooking, place breast side up.
- During last 45 minutes of roasting, remove cover.
- Continue to roast until the leg moves easily and juices run clear.
- Let stand for 20 minutes to let juices settle for easier carving.

FAVORITE MAKEOVER SIDES AND SNACKS

WILD RICE

10 to 12 servings

1 cup wild rice
2 cups water
Salt and pepper to taste

Directions

* In a pan, combine the rice and water.
* Boil, reduce heat and simmer until the rice is tender, usually 40-45 minutes.
* Drain, add seasoning (salt and pepper)

LOW-FAT HUMMUS DIP

10-12 servings

2 cans garbanzo beans drained, and save the juice
6 teaspoons lemon juice
4 tablespoons sesame tahini

6 cloves garlic peeled
1 teaspoon salt
1/2 teaspoon pepper

Directions

* Combine all ingredients in a blender or food processor.
* Process until smooth, and add the reserved garbanzo juice for a nice creamy texture.
* Serve with vegetables. Bell peppers, celery, cucumbers and carrots make a lovely and tasty presentation.
* This recipe makes it possible to prepare two bowls of low-fat hummus, so you can have a presentation in the living room and one in the kitchen while guests keep you company during the turkey preparation.

ACORN SQUASH

10 to 12 servings

5 acorn squash cut in half, scoop out seeds
1/2 cup of water

Directions

- Preheat oven to 350 degrees.
- Put acorn squash halves, cut side down, in a baking pan.
- Add 1/2 cup of water and bake under tender (usually 30-50 minutes)

ENDIVE, WATERCRESS AND PEAR SALAD

10-12 servings

Watercress, 3 large bunches, stems removed
Belgian endive, 3 heads, cored
and separated into leaves
Extra-virgin olive oil, 5 tablespoons

Salt and Ground pepper, to taste
White balsamic vinegar (or pear
vinegar), 3 tablespoons
3 ripe pears, halved and cored, then
cut in half again lengthwise

Directions

- In a large bowl, toss watercress and Belgian endive.
- Add 5 tablespoons of extra-virgin olive oil and toss again.
- Sprinkle salt and freshly ground pepper, toss.
- Pour white balsamic vinegar, or pear vinegar, and then toss.
- Garnish your salad with the pear wedges. Serve immediately.

FAVORITE MAKEOVER DESSERTS

BAKED APPLES

10 to 12 servings
My husband taught me this delicious recipe. It's an old family favorite!

12 tart Jonathon apples
1-1/2 cups brown sugar
12 tablespoons light margarine (Smart Balance Light)
6 teaspoons ground cinnamon

Directions

* Preheat oven to 350 degrees.
* Core the apples but leave the bottom intact, so it looks like a "well" in the apple.
* Prick the apple skins with a fork so the apple can "breathe" while baking.
* Fill the hole with 2 tablespoons of brown sugar and 1 tablespoon of butter substitute.
* Then place the apples in a baking dish with a thin layer of water on the bottom, and sprinkle each apple with cinnamon.
* Bake at 350 degrees for 20 minutes (10 minutes covered with foil and 10 minutes uncovered) until the apples are tender and begin to caramelize.

You can also add chopped walnuts or pecans to the "stuffing". And you may want to top this yummy recipe with a low-fat frozen vanilla yogurt.

Converting to Metrics

VOLUME MEASUREMENT CONVERSIONS

U.S.	Metric
1/4 teaspoon	1.25 ml
1/2 teaspoon	2.5 ml
3/4 teaspoon	3.75 ml
1 teaspoon	5 ml
1 tablespoon	15 ml
1/4 cup	62.5 ml
1/2 cup	125 ml
3/4 cup	187.5 ml
1 cup	250 ml

WEIGHT CONVERSION MEASUREMENTS

U.S.	Metric
1 ounce	28.4 g
8 ounces	227.5 g
16 ounces (1 pound)	455 g

COOKING TEMPERATURE CONVERSIONS

Celsius/Centigrade	0°C and 100°C are arbitrarily placed at the melting and boiling points of water and standard to the metric system
Fahrenheit	Fahrenheit established 0°F as the stabilized temperature when equal amounts of ice, water, and salt are mixed.

To convert temperatures in Fahrenheit to Celsius, use this formula:
$$C = (F-32) \times 0.5555$$
So, for example, if you are baking at 350° F and want to know
that temperature in Celsius, use this calculation:
$$C = (350-32) \times 0.5555 = 176.66°C$$

Chapter 15 You've Just Begun

You have just completed The Menopause Makeover. Congratulations! You have started creating the new you. Do you like what you see? Do you feel good? Is there room for improvement? Was your Makeover so incredible that you want to relax and enjoy your successes? Is it time for another party?

This is the Menopause Makeover debriefing chapter! After you access your Makeover, you have a number of possibilities.

- Repeat the 12-Week Plan with revised goals.
- Repeat the 12-Week Plan with the same goals, so you have extra time to achieve your results.
- Start a support group with other menopausal gals and share your secrets.
- Start a support group and do The Menopause Makeover as a team.
- Share your success story online at www.menopausemakeover.com.

AFTER YOUR MAKEOVER

How Do You Feel After Your Menopause Makeover?

Did you achieve most of your goals? ☐ Yes ☐ No

What specific results did you accomplish?

Overall, in what area(s) did you excel?
Check all that apply:

☐ hormones ☐ nutrition ☐ exercise ☐ beauty

☐ emotions ☐ relationships ☐ spirituality ☐ happiness

What area needs improvement?

Do you need to reset goals? ☐ Yes ☐ No

Were you too ambitious? ☐ Yes ☐ No

Not ambitious enough? ☐ Yes ☐ No

Did you get support from friends and loved ones? ☐ Yes ☐ No

Do you feel prettier after your *Makeover* ☐ Yes ☐ No

Do you feel happier after your *Makeover?* ☐ Yes ☐ No

Do you feel better about your body? ☐ Yes ☐ No

Do you have fewer symptoms? ☐ Yes ☐ No

Are you working closely with your practitioner
to achieve menopausal health? ☐ Yes ☐ No

Did you create an exercise program that you enjoy
and that fits into your lifestyle? ☐ Yes ☐ No

Did you honor your weekly food plans? ☐ Yes ☐ No

What are you most thankful about after completing your *Makeover?*

What relationships improved?

Are your emotions more stable? ☐ N/A ☐ Yes ☐ No

What symptoms still need attention?

What symptoms disappeared?

What new beauty goal are you enjoying most?

Have you grown as a person over the past 12 weeks? ☐ Yes ☐ No

Are you pursuing your goals daily? ☐ Yes ☐ No

What do you enjoy most during the 12-Week Plan?

When you repeat *The Menopause Makeover*, what one thing would you change?

Did You Meet Your Goals for:

Health	☐ Yes	☐ No
Hormones	☐ Yes	☐ No
Nutrition	☐ Yes	☐ No
Exercise	☐ Yes	☐ No
Beauty	☐ Yes	☐ No
Emotions	☐ Yes	☐ No
Relationships	☐ Yes	☐ No
Spirituality	☐ Yes	☐ No
Happiness	☐ Yes	☐ No

Rate Each Area of Your Menopause Makeover – *10, you excelled; 1, no results:*

EXCELLED	10	9	8	7	6	5	4	3	2	1	NO RESULTS
Health	○	○	○	○	○	○	○	○	○	○	Health
Hormones	○	○	○	○	○	○	○	○	○	○	Hormones
Nutrition	○	○	○	○	○	○	○	○	○	○	Nutrition
Exercise	○	○	○	○	○	○	○	○	○	○	Exercise
Beauty	○	○	○	○	○	○	○	○	○	○	Beauty
Emotions	○	○	○	○	○	○	○	○	○	○	Emotions
Relationships	○	○	○	○	○	○	○	○	○	○	Relationships
Spirituality	○	○	○	○	○	○	○	○	○	○	Spirituality
Happiness	○	○	○	○	○	○	○	○	○	○	Happiness
EXCELLED	10	9	8	7	6	5	4	3	2	1	NO RESULTS

How can you improve in each area?
Health

Hormones

Nutrition

Exercise

Beauty

Emotions

Relationships

Spirituality

Happiness

What area is impossible for improvement?

Why?

Are you willing to move forward without improvement in this area?   ☐ Yes ☐ No

Do you need professional support in this area?

What habits do you need to change so you can achieve your goals?

What behavior is holding you back?

How can you change it, so you can achieve your goals?

What lessons did you learn from your Menopause Makeover?

What are you most excited about after completing your Menopause Makeover?

When will you enjoy your Menopause Makeover reward?

REPEATING THE 12-WEEK PLAN AND SETTING NEW GOALS

What results do you want to achieve for the next 12-Week Plan?

Health

Hormones

Nutrition

Exercise

Beauty

Emotions

Relationships

Spirituality

Happiness

If the goals are the same, what will you change to accomplish your goals?

If the goals are different, how will you stay motivated?

What is your greatest hope for the next 12-Week Plan?

What is your greatest fear?

How will you overcome this fear?

Do you need support to be successful? ☐ Yes ☐ No

Who can support you?

What is your action plan for the next 12 weeks?

What reward will you give yourself when you complete the next 12-week plan?

Future Goals

How could your life be better?

Are you willing to make changes to achieve this goal? ☐ Yes ☐ No

Incorporate all future goals into your next Menopause Makeover. The tracking process in the 12-Week Essential Planner can be used to accomplish *all* your goals. You can personalize each 12 weeks to meet your specific goals.

START YOUR OWN MENOPAUSE SUPPORT GROUP

Accountability is one of the strongest motivators for achieving goals. Millions of women are in one of the stages of menopause in the United States. Since you have completed the Menopause Makeover, share your expertise. Begin your very own Menopause Makeover Support Group. Meet once a week to discuss your goals and challenges; share recipes and exercise regimes; seek emotional support. A sisterhood of menopausal women can offer understanding, information, and some much-needed humor. Brainstorming for yourself and each other can be fun. A group of women with something in common can be a powerful force. Embrace your hardships and celebrate your victories.

EACH DAY IS A NEW JOURNEY TOWARD YOUR POWERFUL POTENTIAL.

AUTHOR'S NOTE

GIVING BACK

Doing the Menopause Makeover gave me an unexpected gift. After practicing all eight steps of the Menopause Makeover (health, nutrition, exercise, beauty, emotions, relationships, spirituality and happiness) and applying them to my life, I finally felt whole and complete. This liberating freedom left me asking, "now what?"

Looking to remarkable women, like Oprah Winfrey, for the answer, a life lesson was revealed. It was time to *give back*. Focusing on giving allowed me to add purpose to my life!

Passionate about women's health I decided to support these organizations, because both are making a remarkable difference in women's health.

You too can help these incredible organizations in their mission to advance women's health. We can forge a path with new health options for our daughters. Release your *powerful potential* and make a difference in women's health.

North American Menopause Society (NAMS) the leading nonprofit scientific organization devoted to promoting women's health and quality of life through an understanding of menopause. NAMS is recognized as the preeminent resource on all aspects of menopause to both healthcare providers and the public. They have a useful list of NAMS certified menopause practitioners and the latest news about menopause and hormone therapy.

For more information: http://www.menopause.org/

The Society for Women's Health Research is the nation's only non-profit organization whose mission is to improve the health of all women through research, education and advocacy. The Society encourages the study of sex differences between women and men that affect the prevention, diagnosis and treatment of disease.

For more information: http://swhr.org

Book References can be found online at www.MenopauseMakeover.com

ACKNOWLEDGMENTS

The Menopause Makeover had a five-year gestation period from its creation to becoming a book. This journey would not have been possible without the incredible support of my husband, Michael Becker. He worked tirelessly so I had the freedom to create, research, and write this book. All the while loving me during moments of serious crankiness while going through one of the biggest changes in my life.

I would like to thank my Mom and Dad, Joyce and Stan Jonekos, for teaching me as a child that I could do anything. I never heard, "girls don't do that." I always heard, "go for it!" My brother, Stan Jonekos, always loved me even when I got him in trouble.

This book would not be in your hands without Rick Broadhead, literary agent extraordinaire. I am forever grateful for Rick's incredible support, wisdom and belief in this book, and for securing the perfect publisher.

An enormous thank you to Deb Brody, Executive Editor at Harlequin, who had the vision to see that menopausal women needed a makeover action planner on the bookshelves, and invited *The Menopause Makeover* into the Harlequin non-fiction family for the first edition. Sarah Pelz, Editor at Harlequin, whose editorial advice honored the tone of this book, and who was fun to work with – thank you.

A big thank you to Dr. Wendy Klein for the medical accuracy of this book. Dr. Klein is truly an advocate for women's health, as well as a woman of excellence both personally and professionally.

Speaking of doctors, I must thank my own lifetime doctor, Dr. Josephine Hall. She has been a crusader for my health since I was 20 years old. Had it not been for my own absence from her care, I would not have had the menopause challenges I experienced.

A special thank you to my good friends, Kathryn Hewitt, Terri Seifried, and Sara Martin, who listened to me chatter on and on about menopause and offered their expertise when needed, usually at the last minute. And to my other close gal pals (Colleen, Sheri, Theresa, Sonya, Joan, Nancy, Pamela, Renay and Claire) - going through menopause without a girlfriend is like getting married without a groom – it is just not possible.

Thank you to Lisa Wallender, Judy Morton and Elyssia Stratton for doing *The Menopause Makeover* with great success and inspiring others by sharing their stories.

The 2nd Edition would not be possible without the talent of Stephanee Killen, owner of Intergrative Link. Her enthusiasm and knowledge of the publishing business saved the day!

I would also like to thank Carol Peper, an incredible writer herself, for giving me support and encouragement from the beginning.

And finally, I would like to thank all the women I encountered on my journey who believed in *The Menopause Makeover*.

ABOUT THE AUTHORS

Staness Jonekos is an advocate for women's health, wellness and empowerment. Despite having a name that's derived from the man's name *Stanley*, Staness has been a lifelong crusader for women.

She is an award-winning television writer, producer and director, a published author on women's health, Founder/CEO of Eat Like a Woman® a Nutritional Lifestyle, and one of the original executive producers who launched the television network *Oxygen Media*, co-founded by Oprah Winfrey. Staness delivered five series and co-created Oxygen Media's *Be Fearless* campaign to empower women.

Following her commitment to health, Staness co-executive produced the premiere season of VH1's *Celebrity Fit Club*, and post produced Lifetime's *Speaking of Women's Health*.

Her second book, *Eat Like a Woman and Never Diet Again,* incorporates the latest science in women's health embracing sex differences and how women metabolize food and lose weight differently than men. This book inspired her new brand Eat Like a Woman® a Nutritional Lifestyle.

Staness is a tireless advocate for women's health, wellness, and empowerment. She has appeared on *The Today Show, Fox and Friends, Access Hollywood* and contributes to the *Huffington Post*, and has been featured in a variety of publications from the *Washington Post* to the *Houston Chronicle.*

Ms. Jonekos holds a Bachelor's degree in theater from UCLA and is an active member of the Producers Guild of America, The Academy of Television Arts & Sciences, The North American Menopause Society, and the International Menopause Society.

She lives in Los Angeles with her husband and two pups.

Dr. Wendy Klein is a pioneer and leader in woman's health. Once voted Virginia Commonwealth University's "Woman of the Year," she is an outstanding clinician and scholar who has been repeatedly honored as not just one of the best physicians in her hometown of Richmond, but one of the best doctors in America.

Board-certified in Internal Medicine, she is an Associate Professor Emeritus of Medicine, Obstetrics and Gynecology at Virginia Commonwealth University School of Medicine. She co-founded the Women's Health Center at Stony Point, where she served as Medical Director. Dr. Klein also established the unique Women's Health Residency Program at VCU, which has been lauded as one of the best programs of its kind in the United States.

As co-founder of the Association of Academic Women's Health Programs, a national consortium of women's health educators, clinicians and researchers, the founder of the annual VCU Women's Health Update Continuing Medical Education Conference, one of the premier women's health conferences in the country, and the founder of the Women in Medicine, Science and Dentistry Organization (WISDM), Dr. Klein is committed to advancing women's health through education.

She is former deputy editor of the Journal of Women's Health, past co-chair of the VCU School of Medicine's Committee on the Status of Women and Minorities, senior deputy director emeritus of the Virginia Commonwealth University Institute for Women's Health, a National Center for Excellence, and past gubernatorial appointee to both the Virginia Council on the Status of Women and the Governor's Task Force on Cervical Cancer. She currently serves on the Virginia Board of Health.

Dr. Klein received the Leadership Award from the Institute for the Advancement of Multicultural and Minority Medicine, and was honored by the VCU faculty as the recipient of the annual WISDM Professional Achievement Award. An active member and contributor to the North American Menopause Society and a Master of the American College of Physicians, Dr. Klein enthusiastically lectures on hormone therapy, osteoporosis and women's health, midlife and beyond. At this time, she is medical director of the Fan Free Clinic in Richmond, Virginia.

Married for over 25 years to the man of her dreams, Dr. Klein lives in Richmond, Virginia and is the mother of two children of whom she is exceedingly proud.

Fitness Blender
Low impact Cardio Workout for Beginners
30:04

CPSIA information can be obtained
at www.ICGtesting.com
Printed in the USA
LVOW03s1822240716
497581LV00029B/917/P